Contents

Out of the Maze

REACHING AND SUPPORTING LONDONERS WITH SEVERE MENTAL HEALTH PROBLEMS

ANGELA GREATLEY WITH RICHARD FORD

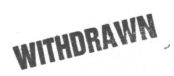

The King's Fund
The King's Fund is an independent charitable foundation working for better health, especially in London. We carry out research, policy analysis and development activities, working on our own, in partnerships, and through grants. We are a major resource to people working in health, offering leadership and education courses; seminars and workshops; publications; information and library services; a specialist bookshop; and conference and meeting facilities.

Charity registration number: 207401

The Sainsbury Centre for Mental Health
The Sainsbury Centre for Mental Health is a registered charity, working to improve the quality of life for people with severe mental health problems. It aims to influence national policy and encourage good practice in mental health services, through a coordinated programme of research, training and development. The Centre is affiliated to King's College London.

A charitable company limited by guarantee. Registered in England and Wales number: 4373019. Charity registration number: 1091156

Published by

King's Fund
11–13 Cavendish Square
London W1G 0AN
www.kingsfund.org.uk

The Sainsbury Centre for Mental Health
134–138 Borough High Street
London SE1 1LB
www.scmh.org.uk

ISBN 1 85717 469 0

A CIP catalogue record for this book is available from the British Library

Available from

King's Fund Bookshop
11–13 Cavendish Square
London W1G 0AN
Tel: 020 7307 2591
Fax: 020 7307 2801
www.kingsfundbookshop.org.uk

The Sainsbury Centre for Mental Health
134–138 Borough High Street
London SE1 1LB
Tel: 020 7827 8300
Fax: 020 7403 9482
www.scmh.org.uk

Edited by Alan Dingle
Cover design by Minuche Mazumdar Farrar
Typeset by Grasshopper Design Company
Printed and bound in Great Britain

Acknowledgements

The teams

We would like to thank the managers, the staff, the clients and their carers from the three Working Together in London teams: Antenna in Haringey, the Islington Assertive Outreach Team and the Lambeth Early Onset team. All tackled the development programme with great enthusiasm and have been willing to share their findings very widely.

The Funders' Group

We owe an enormous debt of thanks to the members of the Funders' Group, who developed this programme and supported it throughout. The members were:

Professor Elaine Murphy (Chair of the group)
Mrs Susan Elizabeth (Director of Grants, The King's Fund, until 2001)
Dr Paul O'Halloran (Director of Training and Practice Development, The Sainsbury Centre for Mental Health)
Mr Martin Brown (Department of Health)
Ms Elaine Edgar (Department of Health)
Ms Elaine Best (Department of Health)
Dr Matt Muijen (Chief Executive, The Sainsbury Centre for Mental Health)
Rabbi Julia Neuberger (Chief Executive, The King's Fund)
Mrs Janice Robinson (Director, Health and Social Care Programme, The King's Fund)

We would also like to thank Lord Hunt of King's Heath for the encouragement he gave to the development of the programme and for his support in the early stages.

The evaluation team

Those who contributed to the evaluation were:

- *Core team:* John Lee, Paul McCrone, Richard Ford
- *Design, data collection and analysis:* Edana Minghella, Helen Scott, Ganesh Sathyamoorthy
- *Design and data collection:* Ahmed Agha, Mike Barnett, Loren Buckley, John O'Brien, David Pearce, Maki Spanoudis, Angela Sweeney, Neoklis Veniamin
- *Interviewer training:* Debbie Mayes, Sarah Lewis, Nutan Kotecha, Brigid Morris, Graeme Kerr, Sian Taylder

We are also grateful to all the staff of the King's Fund and the Sainsbury Centre for Mental Health who contributed to the development programme and to this review.

Angela Greatley and Richard Ford

Executive summary

"The team has brought me a better understanding of mental illness and I feel able to deal with it. Before I ignored it and I wasn't able to deal with it, and I didn't want to accept help."

Lambeth client

The background

The care of people with severe and long-term mental health problems who do not want to use, or 'engage' with, services presents a major challenge. They may not get the treatment they need. They often have additional problems with money, housing, employment, education and training. Some also have problems of substance misuse. As a result, they may experience social exclusion. People from some black and minority ethnic communities are fearful of mental health services and may be more excluded. Assertive outreach services have been shown to be effective in helping people with these problems.

Assertive outreach is a way of organising intensive, user-centred community mental health care and support for people with severe problems who will not readily engage with services. Assertive outreach has become a central plank of mental health policy. After brief references in the *National Service Framework for Mental Health*, interest in and commitment to developing the approach increased. Assertive outreach was named as a key component of community mental health policy in the *NHS Plan* and its importance was emphasised in *The Mental Health Policy Implementation Guide*.

The Working Together in London programme was set up by the King's Fund, the Sainsbury Centre for Mental Health and the Department of Health to establish assertive outreach teams and develop new ways of working that can bring about the social inclusion of people with severe and long-term mental health problems, by helping them to find housing, work and a social network.

The teams

The programme supported the setting up of three pilot teams – the Antenna service in Haringey, the Islington Assertive Outreach Team and Lambeth Early Onset – that would use the assertive outreach approach to help this difficult-to-reach client group.

The teams in this study also formed partnerships with other organisations within and outside the mental health field, so that the benefits might be felt not just by the programme's clients but also by anyone with mental health problems locally.

Antenna Outreach Service, Haringey

The Antenna assertive outreach team in north London provides a culturally sensitive mental health service to young people from African and Caribbean communities, with staff recruited from the communities. The service offers support and advice to families and other carers. It works beyond the boundaries of mental health services to help young people with serious mental health problems to achieve a better quality of life.

Islington Assertive Outreach Team

The Islington team, also in north London, works with an older group of clients who have experienced serious problems over a long period. Working with dual diagnosis is a particular feature of the team's work and links are being forged with the wide variety of minority ethnic communities living in the area.

Lambeth Early Onset

Lambeth Early Onset (LEO), in south London, provides services to a younger group of clients who have already experienced the onset of severe mental health problems. The team works to reduce the trauma of contact with mental health services and, by working closely with education and employment, aims to promote recovery. User and carer groups are a particular feature of the team's work.

The effectiveness of the teams was assessed by researchers from the Sainsbury Centre for Mental Health and the Centre for the Economics of Mental Health.

The researchers asked a range of local stakeholders for their views on the programme. Service users of the three teams were also asked for their views on the assertive outreach services.

Findings

Tackling social exclusion

On many occasions, service users were able to give examples of how they had been helped with housing, employment, education, leisure, religion, benefits and with their family relationships. These are all areas that are central to social inclusion. Users said that they felt better, not just in terms of their mental health, but also about their lives in general.

Developing sustainable partnerships

The review shows that new partnerships are needed if services working with people who experience serious and long-term problems are to be able to help them gain a better quality of life. However, these partnerships are not easy to forge and sustain. Mental health services have to prioritise the development of new partnerships if they are to make a lasting difference for service users.

Integrating new services

New services cannot be introduced without significant impact on existing services. Failure to deal with the potential impact of new developments may mean that new services struggle to work in the most effective way. Assertive outreach services deal with a very specific group of users but must be integrated with other community health and in-patient services.

Implementing key success factors

The Government has determined that there should be 220 teams by April 2003; therefore many localities are currently developing their assertive outreach services. The review shows that there are key factors for success in developing these new services: multi-disciplinary teams are needed, working with a team-based approach but specialist inputs are also needed. A balance between the medical and social approaches is needed, and all teams must respond to cultural diversity.

Assertive outreach teams that offer a balance of the medical and social approach, that take an active role in promoting inclusion and that work in close collaboration with other health and social care services can help their clients to become more independent and able to cope. Assertive outreach is an important component of a mental health service system.

The recommendations

The report concludes with recommendations for policy-makers and service providers on the following themes:

Promoting the social inclusion of people with mental health problems

Standard 1 of the National Service Framework concerns mental health promotion and combating discrimination; it has provided an important impetus to tackling exclusion, but it is still limited in scope:
- Developing partnerships with local agencies outside the mental health field must be specified as part of the mainstream work of mental health services.
- Commissioners should give priority to developing and sustaining partnerships with housing agencies, welfare benefits service and advice agencies, and education and training providers.
- Partnership working must be properly resourced and there should be a dedicated community development worker in each assertive outreach team.

Working in partnership with the community

Community support can make the work of mental health services more acceptable:
- Mental health services need to engage with community groups and offer them support – information, training and joint working – as well as grant aid; this is particularly important for people from black and minority ethnic communities.
- Mental health problems are particularly common in deprived communities, and therefore mental health agencies will often be operating in the same neighbourhoods as urban regeneration programmes and neighbourhood development schemes. Mental health services need to participate in the planning and implementation of these schemes, both to advance the interests of people with known mental health problems and to promote new ways of thinking about mental health in the community.

- Spirituality and religious observance are known to be very important to many people with severe mental health problems. Mental health services should therefore aim to form partnerships with faith communities, which may have their own support systems for people with such problems.

Establishing and maintaining assertive outreach teams

Plans to set up new teams should be realistic if the considerable investment they represent is not to be lost by failure at a later stage.

Trusts should:
- Allocate time and resources for recruitment and team training.
- Provide development support for both new and existing teams.
- Recruit from a range of disciplines initially, but re-balance skills and experience within the team as it works towards meeting the needs of its target group.

Assertive outreach teams:
- Must be able to offer a full range of bio-psycho-social interventions if clients are to engage with services, receive high-quality and up-to-date treatment and improve their quality of life.
- May need additional specialist resources (such as in dual diagnosis) to complement, rather than replace, the work of other team members.
- Should work to prescribed standards, but can adapt their approach to conform to local cultural norms.
- Should have a clear understanding about the balance between the medical and the social approaches and about team organisation if their staff are to achieve sustainable working arrangements.

Achieving a more integrated system of mental health services

Assertive outreach teams should give early priority to forming working relationships with existing mental health services (including in-patient teams), with other new teams (such as crisis resolution) and with primary care. They should aim to develop an approach that will, over time, reduce reliance on expensive in-patient beds for crisis admissions and for lengthy hospital stays:
- A local communications programme is needed early on to advise on the functions and potential of any new teams – assertive outreach, crisis resolution or early intervention – and on how their work will relate to existing services.
- Arrangements for referral and for the acceptance of clients must be agreed with existing services: in particular, the speed and nature of the referral process.
- Assertive outreach teams must monitor the use of in-patient beds by their clients and plan to change the nature of these admissions over time.
- The possible effects of research intervention need to be assessed at the beginning of a programme and explained within the mental health system. Monitoring systems should identify unintended effects so that these can be tackled.
- In order to maximise referrals from primary care, assertive outreach teams will need to explain to primary care trusts what their role, functions and potential are.

Introduction

I feel fine now . . . I'm feeling more independent. I couldn't see a future for myself but I can see the next five to seven years ahead now.

Emotionally I feel strong and the team was there for me . . . All in all I feel I have got stronger and stronger.

I feel more independent and able to cope. The team make me more independent . . . I think they are doing a lot of good things.

These optimistic comments come from the clients of three pilot assertive outreach teams – Antenna in Haringey, Islington Assertive Outreach and Lambeth Early Onset – that target people in London with serious and long-term mental health problems who do not use services.

The teams are part of the Working Together in London programme, a three-year, £2 million initiative jointly organised by the King's Fund, the Sainsbury Centre for Mental Health and the Department of Health. The aim of the programme, which began its work in 1998, is to develop integrated, community-based support services for people with severe mental health problems.

Many deprived communities, especially in London, experience very high rates of mental illness, but previous mental health services were often overstretched or badly targeted. In designing the Working Together in London programme, the organisers took particular account of the fact that people with serious and long-term mental health problems often have difficulty in:

- finding the right kind of treatment and care
- sustaining a decent quality of life
- getting and keeping a home.

As a result, they often live in poverty and isolation, with few friends and support networks. They often go from one service to another, getting only a partial response from each.

For people from London's black and minority ethnic communities, these difficulties are magnified. There are high rates of compulsory treatment, particularly for young men from African and Caribbean communities, and growing mental health problems among young Asian, women. The options for treatment and care are limited: although there are some voluntary sector initiatives, it is hard for people from black and minority ethnic communities to find the support they need to maintain a decent quality of life.

These are all problems of *social exclusion*, and it was clear that a new approach was needed. The Working Together in London programme set out to create more integrated service responses to meet the complex needs of people with long-term and serious mental health problems. It hoped to bring improvements to a wider range of service users in an area and not just to the clients of the new teams.

The Working Together in London programme had three explicit aims:

1. to set up assertive outreach teams that would meet the needs of people with serious and long-term mental health problems
2. to promote the social inclusion of people with severe mental illness
3. to achieve better integration of local mental health services.

This report examines the work of the three pilot teams, drawing out the key lessons for health and social work professionals and offering practical guidelines on how to put assertive outreach into practice. Its target audience includes: health commissioners in primary care trusts; mental health providers and policy makers in both national and local government; and voluntary sector organisations that support people with mental illness.

The first part of the report describes the context in which the three teams operate:

- the history of the Working Together in London programme
- the history of assertive outreach
- social exclusion and mental health
- regeneration and mental health
- faith communities and mental health.

The second part of the report gives detailed case studies of the three teams, describing:

- what previous mental health services were like in their area
- how the new teams were set up
- what kind of service they offer
- their successes and their problems.

The third part of the report deals with opportunities for broader change, describing:

- mental health services and regeneration issues
- mental health services and faith communities.

Part four of the report gives the views of local stakeholders on how the teams operated. This is followed by a set of conclusions and recommendations for service providers and policy makers.

Comments by clients of the three teams are distributed throughout the text. Case studies written by the project teams showing some of the real-life problems experienced by clients have also been included. Clients' names have been changed throughout.

Note: throughout this report the term 'service user(s)' is used to describe anyone who uses or has tried to use any specialist mental health service. The word 'clients' is reserved for people who have been using the services of the three teams being studied.

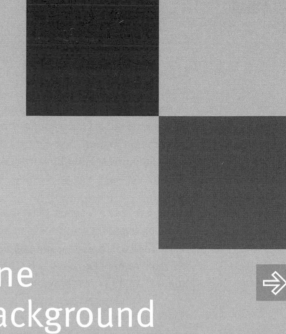

Part one
The background

The report begins by looking at the origins of the Working
Together in London programme: the policy environment, the
sponsors, the people the programme targeted, how the
participants were chosen and how they were supported.

There follows a brief introduction to the assertive outreach
approach, describing its beginnings in the USA, the core
elements needed to make it a success, and the continuing
debate about the importance of 'fidelity to the model'.

Next, the importance of ensuring the social inclusion of
people with severe mental health problems is highlighted.
Social exclusion partly results from poor housing,
unemployment and a lack of education and training, and
therefore is best tackled by broad partnerships of agencies,
both from within the mental health system and outside.

→ CASE STUDY: DAVID

David is 20 years old, single and lives with his family. At 17 he had his first contact with mental health services. Following an interview with a counsellor, he was formally assessed and found to have psychotic symptoms. After an informal overnight admission to a local acute hospital ward, he and his family decided he should go home. Soon afterwards, David was seen by a local community mental health team, but he rarely attended appointments, and didn't take – or even collect – his prescription for anti-psychotic medication. About seven months after this first admission, his mother took him back to the team because his behaviour had deteriorated and was increasingly difficult for the family to manage.

This led to David's second hospital admission – this time under the Mental Health Act – lasting five months. The assertive outreach team became involved and plans were made to discharge him from hospital, using the Care Programme Approach. David and his family were seen weekly by the team, who discussed his problems, the recent admission, and how things could move forward for him.

David wanted to work. He got a job but struggled to cope. The long hours meant that he was often tired and he started to take his tablets intermittently. After two months he was relapsing. Although David denied any problems, his family reported early signs of relapsing. These signs had been identified earlier with David and his family, and a plan had been agreed to manage them. David continued to deny his problems but team visits and discussions were increased to provide support for him and his family.

As problems became more pronounced, there was increasing tension in the family home, with arguments and damage to property. The team started to visit every day to offer support and to ensure that David was following his prescription. The relapse lasted about three months but admission to hospital was avoided.

David slowly recovered, and efforts were made to help him find work or training and to find independent accommodation. He completed a pre-employment training course, and was interviewed successfully for supported housing. He has now recovered fully from his relapse and hasn't had to go into hospital.

The team's approach shows how the assertive outreach approach was extremely effective. The team offered a seven-day-a-week service, combined with assertive outreach interventions, using a psychosocial model: helping David to explore and gain employment and training, and housing. They worked with family support and with David to help him understand his illness, and to learn skills to cope with it. The work that the team did to gain his trust, and help him through his relapse, was essential to this positive outcome.

1 The Working Together in London programme

The policy environment

Assertive outreach has become a central plank of mental health policy. After brief references in the *National Service Framework for Mental Health* (Department of Health, 1999), interest in the approach increased, and it was named as an essential element of community mental health care in the *NHS Plan* (Department of Health, 2000) and *The Mental Health Policy Implementation Guide* (Department of Health, 2001). The challenge is to devise the kind of treatment and care that people will use and to provide it in the areas of highest need. Assertive outreach is examined in detail in chapter 2.

The stimulus for the Working Together in London programme was a group of pioneering reports published in the late 1990s by the programme's organisers.

The King's Fund

In 1997 the King's Fund published *London's mental health*, a major investigation by leading mental health academics and practitioners which concluded that current mental health services 'cannot be sustained' and that no single service had 'a full range of desirable features' (Johnson, 1997).

Transforming health in London, a subsequent report by the King's Fund London Commission, found that:

> There is a new generation of young and middle aged Londoners with serious mental illness who have never received care in long-stay psychiatric institutions. Though in need of long-term care and support, the hostels, group homes, congregate day centres and work schemes developed for people resettled from the old asylums do not find favour with them. They seek more individualised approaches . . . Suitable care packages are difficult to organise, with the result that repeated short admissions to acute psychiatric beds necessarily become the pattern of care.
>
> King's Fund, 1997

The report went on to say that new forms of care, including assertive outreach, might be more helpful but were lacking throughout most of the capital.

The Sainsbury Centre for Mental Health (SCMH)

The Sainsbury Centre for Mental Health (SCMH) was also exploring new ways of helping people with the most serious problems in the most deprived urban areas. Its review *Keys to engagement* (Sainsbury Centre for Mental Health, 1998) noted the progress made in mental health care over the preceding thirty years, but said that it is often 'the most vulnerable who receive the least appropriate care'. This review also recommended the wider use of assertive outreach in British mental health care.

The Department of Health

The Department of Health was also keen to promote new ways of supporting people with serious, long-term mental health problems. In 1998 it published *Modernising mental health* (Department of Health, 1998), which spoke of creating a service that was 'safe, sound and supportive'. This subsequently led to the publication of the *National Service Framework for Mental Health* (Department of Health, 1999).

Figure 1 sets out the way the programme was designed.

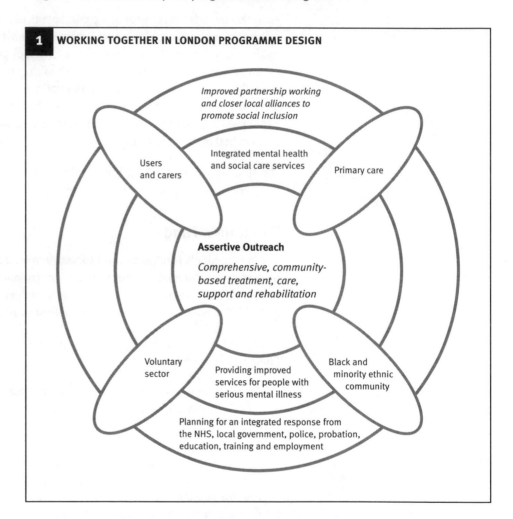

1 WORKING TOGETHER IN LONDON PROGRAMME DESIGN

Improved partnership working and closer local alliances to promote social inclusion

Integrated mental health and social care services

Users and carers

Primary care

Assertive Outreach

Comprehensive, community-based treatment, care, support and rehabilitation

Voluntary sector

Providing improved services for people with serious mental illness

Black and minority ethnic community

Planning for an integrated response from the NHS, local government, police, probation, education, training and employment

Who is the programme trying to help?

When I have a crisis – I've had a few, eight or nine incidences of being ill in the last three or four years – it's always been dealt with by me going to hospital, being evaluated and then going in, but recently I've been able to calm myself down and the team helped with that . . . I've talked to the team a lot about what a well balanced state is and how to find stability and how to be happy and friendly with people.

Islington interviewee

Some people have mental health problems of such intensity that they are unable to function adequately within their own culture and environment. These problems are often long term, lasting at least twelve months and sometimes much longer. Minghella, Gauntlett and Ford (2002) examined the diagnoses for assertive outreach clients in two well-established British teams: the most common diagnosis was schizophrenia, with smaller percentages experiencing other psychotic illnesses.

Some of the people in this group will have had many hospital admissions – often compulsory – and seem destined to have many more in the future. They often live chaotic lives, struggling to manage their money, their home and their relationships. However good the treatment and however careful the discharge planning, people with this range of problems may quickly relapse without intensive support to maintain their quality of life.

The lives of people with serious and long-term mental illness can be further complicated by the use of alcohol and illicit drugs (Drake *et al*, 2001). They often have difficulty in finding a home – and even if they do get somewhere to live, they may have problems in maintaining it and may become homeless again. They are often desperately poor. Their lives are at risk from suicide and self-harm, and they suffer the rejection and prejudice of a society that fears mentally ill people.

People with this range of problems may be suspicious of mental health services. Some may have experienced poor quality mental health care in the past, including compulsory admissions. Some may have been in local authority care when younger; others may have been in prisons or other institutions. The idea of seeking help voluntarily, turning up for appointments and following prescribed treatments, is alien to them. They simply refuse to engage with services.

There are additional deterrents for people from black and minority ethnic communities. They may have been hospitalised on a compulsory basis; members of some communities still experience higher rates of admission under compulsion. They may have heard about the experiences of other black people in the mental health system and have decided to avoid it. Here are the words of a service user quoted in *Breaking the circles of fear: a review of the relationship between mental health services and African and Caribbean communities* (Sainsbury Centre for Mental Health, 2002):

> *Coming to mental health services was like the last straw . . . you come to services disempowered already, they strip you of your dignity . . . you become the dregs of society.*

How many people?

The target group for the Working Together in London programme is small: in 1998 the Sainsbury Centre for Mental Health estimated that there were perhaps fifteen thousand people with this range of problems at any one time (Sainsbury Centre for Mental Health, 1998) and the *NHS Plan* suggests that there may be twenty thousand (Department of Health, 2000). However, people with serious mental health problems are disproportionately represented in poorer urban areas. A deprived inner city area might need to provide an assertive outreach service for about 200 per 100,000 of the adult population aged 16–64, whereas the requirement will be much less in a wealthier suburban area.

Working towards social inclusion

There has long been debate about how best to organise care and treatment for people with serious and long-term mental health problems. Years ago, many of them would have lived out their lives within the narrow confines of Victorian asylums. Today they can receive the best treatment and care outside institutions – but for the reasons given above, they are often suspicious of such services.

The Victorian asylums did more than just provide treatment. They also provided food, shelter, activities and sometimes work – however poor the quality of life. Although over the past fifty years people with serious and long-term mental health problems have been treated with increasing success in the community, sufficient attention has not always been given to their needs for decent housing, leisure activities, work and ordinary friendships.

They need that extra support if they are to lead the sort of lives that we all want. People with serious mental health problems will often speak more about their need for support than about their need for treatment. They want a home, some money in their pocket or purse, something interesting to do during the day – including the chance to go out to work – and friends.

In responding to a 1999 Mind inquiry, a service user summed up the situation as follows:

> *Social inclusion must come down to somewhere to live, something to do, someone to love. It's as simple – and as complicated – as that. There are all kinds of barriers to people with mental health problems having those three things.*

> Dunn, 1999

Improvements for all

Community mental health services acknowledge these needs and try to help service users achieve a better quality of life. But working at the level of the individual can be of limited value: mental health services should also help to improve the circumstances of everyone who experiences severe mental health problems. And because so many people live disadvantaged lives, mental health must work alongside other public services to bring about improvements.

Assertive outreach has a specific role to play in tackling the problems experienced by clients with the most serious and long-term problems, where disadvantage and poverty combine with long-term prejudice and stigma to create social exclusion.

> *People with significant mental illness are amongst the most excluded in society.*

> Sayce and Measey, 1999

The Working Together in London programme was designed to tackle exclusion and work for inclusion, although these terms were less widely used in 1998 when it began work. The programme was designed to see how far the new assertive outreach teams could change key services outside the immediate world of mental health. The aim was to establish what the teams could contribute to bringing about the social inclusion of people with mental health problems, whether they were clients of the assertive outreach teams or the users of other services.

How the programme was set up

The Working Together in London programme was set up with a budget of £2 million, which the organisers decided would be spent in three areas of the capital. They told mental health services across London that the new programme was starting up and invited them to bid for the opportunity to take part in it.

Only broadly based consortiums were eligible to bid. These groups were to form the nucleus of the steering groups that would see the programme through. In order to test local commitment, the groups had to include representatives of all stakeholders: the commissioners and providers – both statutory and voluntary – of mental health and social care, black and minority ethnic groups and local users, all of whom had to be in support of a proposal.

The organisers received fourteen proposals from would-be steering groups and in autumn 1998 chose three of them, based in Haringey, Islington and Lambeth respectively. The new teams, set up in 1999, each received funding to provide an assertive outreach service for two years, plus development funding for exploring how to improve the social inclusion of people with the most serious mental health problems.

The organisers also commissioned an evaluation of the programme from a group of researchers at the Sainsbury Centre for Mental Health and the Centre for the Economics of Mental Health. This evaluation would not focus on assertive outreach itself – a great deal of research has already been done into that topic (see chapter 2) – but on the integration of mental health services, the development of partnerships and service user costs. Most importantly, the researchers would try to find out what the users thought of assertive outreach services. The Sainsbury User Focused Monitoring Team was to carry out this part of the evaluation: in other words, users would interview users. Rather than place the comments of the users all together in a single chapter – which seemed to us a form of segregation – we have distributed them throughout the text of the book to demonstrate the importance of their comments.

Recruiting and training the teams

The Sainsbury Centre for Mental Health had agreed to provide 'hands-on' training for each of the teams as it came into being. A member of the SCMH staff experienced in delivering assertive outreach was therefore allocated to each site. But the first job was to recruit the workers who would make up the teams.

As soon as it had been selected, each team received some of the grant aid to enable it to recruit staff. But even at this stage it was clear that the setting up of the new teams would have implications for other parts of the mental health services. Some staff left existing teams to join the new service and this created difficulties locally. For Lambeth, recruitment came at a time when mental health services were being reorganised following the creation of the new South London and Maudsley Trust; as a result, all staff felt uncertain about their future. Recruitment to LEO was slow as people took their time to think about whether to join the new venture. However, all of the teams were functioning by the end of 1999 and the Sainsbury Centre for Mental Health had provided the initial package of team training.

Maintaining support for the programme

New health and social care services sometimes fail to thrive because local managers, clinicians, community groups and users do not feel that they 'own' them. The organisers knew that if the three new teams were to succeed they needed not just funding, but also local champions. Fortunately, the steering groups in all three areas maintained their enthusiastic support for the teams and their development work. Hence the success of the Working Together in London programme is due not simply to the hard work of the assertive outreach staff but also to the commitment of the local people who collaborated with them.

The programme was formally launched in 1998 by Lord Hunt of King's Heath and was later led by Professor Elaine Murphy, chair of the Funders' Group, which represented the King's Fund, the Sainsbury Centre for Mental Health and the Department of Health. The Working Together in London programme was fortunate to enjoy the enthusiastic support of this group, committed to improving mental health care and support services for some of the most deprived people in London.

Summary

- Assertive outreach has come to be regarded as 'an essential element of community mental health care'.
- The Working Together in London programme was set up by the King's Fund, the Sainsbury Centre for Mental Health and the Department of Health to use assertive outreach to support people with severe and long-term mental health problems who do not use services.
- People with severe and long-term mental health problems tend to experience a range of parallel problems with (for example) money, housing, employment, education/training and substance abuse. As a result, they often suffer from social exclusion.
- People from black and minority ethnic (BME) communities tend to suffer disproportionately from these problems, and in addition receive less adequate treatment from existing mental health services than the general population.
- The Working Together in London programme aimed to bring about the social inclusion of people with severe and long-term mental health problems by helping them to find housing, a job and a social network.
- The programme operated by forming partnerships with other organisations inside and outside the mental health field, so that the benefits might be felt not just by the programme's clients but also by anyone with mental health problems locally.
- The programme invited consortiums of organisations from all over London to bid for the opportunity to set up three pilot assertive outreach teams. The eventual choices were the Antenna service in Haringey, the Islington Assertive Outreach Team and Lambeth Early Onset (LEO).
- Each team was supported by a steering group of people from local organisations.
- The effectiveness of the teams was assessed by researchers from the Sainsbury Centre for Mental Health and the Centre for the Economics of Mental Health.

2 What is assertive outreach?

Assertive outreach is a way of organising intensive, user-centred community mental health care and support for people with long-term and serious problems who will not use services. It is not a specific treatment in itself, but a vehicle for delivering a range of different treatments and interventions.

Assertive outreach is a specialist service, offering an effective way of working with a small and well-defined client group. It should always be targeted at the people who can derive most benefit from it. As with other mental health services, one size cannot be made to fit all: the needs of individual users must determine the service response that will be the most effective and acceptable.

When did assertive outreach begin?

Assertive outreach is a term used primarily in British mental health care. It derives from a model known as 'assertive community treatment' (ACT) – or 'training in community living' as it was initially known. ACT was developed and documented in the mid-1970s by a group of mental health professionals working in Madison, Wisconsin, USA (Dixon, 2000). They saw it as a way of working in the community with people who had hitherto been long-term patients in the psychiatric in-patient services of large institutions.

Mental health services in several countries had been treating people at home rather than in hospital since the middle of the twentieth century. Many clients received high-quality care in these outpatient settings, whether from community mental health teams and centres or from professionals working in individual practices. However, ACT differed in taking a comprehensive approach to the treatment and support of a specific group of people with very severe problems.

Research into the pioneering ACT programme in Wisconsin showed very favourable outcomes for effectiveness, costs and the 'burden' on family and carers (Phillips *et al*, 2001). These positive results led to the adoption of the ACT approach in other areas of North America and in Australia – where the teams were first known as mobile community treatment teams – and in a more limited way in British mental health services. ACT itself became known as the Programme of Assertive Community Treatment (PACT) in many areas. But whatever the term used to describe it, this is essentially an intensive service offered by a team working together to deliver treatment, care and support.

Research into assertive outreach

Research into assertive community treatment and assertive outreach has continued up to the present day in many countries:

> *Never before has a clinical service delivery system been so carefully scrutinised: ACT is the most empirically studied of all community mental health program approaches in existence today.*
> Stein and Santos, 1998

The review *Keys to engagement* (Sainsbury Centre for Mental Health, 1998) looked at the pioneering assertive outreach schemes operating in Britain at that time and concluded that assertive outreach was the right way 'to engage and maintain engagement' with the small group of people with mental health problems who did not readily use services. The study also introduced into Britain the term 'assertive outreach' for assertive community treatment.

In 1998, the Cochrane review by Marshall and Lockwood provided a sound evidence base (Marshall and Lockwood, 1998), and research into the effectiveness of the approach continues. Two of the project teams involved in the Working Together in London programme set up randomised controlled trials (RCTs); the findings will be published in 2003. The pan-London study of assertive outreach teams began work in 2000 and is planning to start publishing its findings in 2004. The National Institute of Mental Health for England is setting up a research network of collaborators to commission NHS research and development, and a further study of assertive outreach is one of its first pieces of work.

Although we shall not be reviewing this ever-growing body of research in this report, it is worth asking why so much of it is still going on when there is already plenty of evidence for the effectiveness of assertive outreach. As we shall see, British researchers have unanswered questions about the transferability of the approach from one country to another and the effects on it of environmental factors.

What does assertive outreach involve?

Assertive outreach offers comprehensive, community-based treatment, rehabilitation and support, delivered by a team largely made up of professionally qualified mental health staff. In some (but not all) teams there are also members who bring a broad range of complementary skills and experience – including that of using mental health services – but do not have a professional qualification. The precise make-up of a team varies according to local circumstances and the attitudes of those setting it up. The three Working Together in London teams each took a slightly different approach, but they all adhered to the basic formula of broadly based multi-professional working.

Keys to engagement pointed out that, although there had been variations in the application of assertive outreach in Britain to date – in, for example, the composition of the team and the way it operated – there was general agreement on the users most likely to benefit from the approach. The Sainsbury study also listed the key elements in effective assertive outreach teams; the

Working Together in London programme offered an opportunity to refine this list further.

There has been considerable debate about the importance of 'fidelity to the model' of assertive outreach: in other words, 'conformity with prescribed elements' of programmes that have proved successful in practice (McGrew *et al*, 1994). Commentators have looked at how closely teams have adhered to the model described in the literature and at how far their success – or failure – is related to the level of fidelity; the claim has been made that 'If you don't do it right, it won't work'.

The debate was conducted in the pages of *The British Journal of Psychiatry* at the same time as the Working Together in London programme was getting started. In 1998 several articles in the journal had described the PriSM study, questioning whether the long-term improvement in the social functioning and symptoms of clients of assertive outreach was any greater than for clients of standard services in ordinary practice in the British context (Thornicroft *et al*, 1998). A year later, the journal carried further articles that in turn cast doubt on whether the PriSM study had actually been looking at properly established assertive outreach in Britain (see, amongst other criticisms, Marshall *et al*, 1999). Throughout the life of the Working Together in London programme, the debate about fidelity has continued.

However, our evaluation of the programme was not designed to explore the question of fidelity but rather to see how the broad assertive outreach approach might develop in some of the most deprived communities in London. We used earlier research and the findings of *Keys to engagement* (Sainsbury Centre for Mental Health, 1998) as our basis, and were more concerned with looking at how new services can be introduced and how the teams developed. Subsequent chapters of this book look at these questions in turn.

Some criteria for assertive outreach

Although they wished to avoid rigid definitions, the teams chosen to take part in Working Together in London all agreed to work to a limited number of criteria. These were based on the recommendations of *Keys to engagement* (Sainsbury Centre for Mental Health, 1998) and can be summarised as follows:

- The team targets only people with severe and enduring illness who do not use other services.
- The service is as intensive and frequent as needed by the client. Visits to individuals can, if necessary, be lengthy and very frequent.
- The team engages with the client on his or her own territory and follows up contacts assertively: for example, it may visit clients at home, meet them in the café or the park or talk to them on the street.
- The team is able to offer a response to a client day or night and every day of the year. Very few teams provide their own cover, in fact, but instead work extended hours and make arrangements with other professionals: for example, with home treatment and crisis resolution.
- The team works long term with the client and does not have a short, predetermined time scale for delivery of the service.
- The team works with family, carers and other people within the client's own support system.

In order to meet these requirements, an assertive outreach team must possess certain characteristics:

- Team members can deliver a range of bio-psycho-social interventions; the team itself originates these interventions, and team members offer most of the treatment, care and support.
- It is multi-disciplinary, with input from a psychiatrist.
- It is a managed team, not a group of individual practitioners operating from the same office.
- It has small caseloads – 1 to 10 is preferred and 1 to 15 is the absolute maximum.
- An entirely new team is set up, with team training and a gradual build-up of clients to enable it to deal effectively with the intensity of demand from each new user.

Those who go on to read the international literature on assertive outreach will realise that the above list of desirable characteristics is a comparatively short one.

The Working Together in London teams that are the subject of this report met all the criteria on the above lists. In addition, ethnicity was an important issue for all the teams; in fact, the Haringey team focused exclusively on African and Caribbean communities. However, this was an extension of the principles of assertive outreach work and was entirely consistent with the approach that had been agreed when the programme was designed.

Fidelity to the model

Some problems over 'fidelity' did emerge, and teams are still considering how best to tackle them.

The team approach versus the keyworker approach

One of the key debates has concerned the relative merits of the keyworker approach and the team approach.

Everyone who has been in touch with specialist mental health services must be registered on the Care Programme Approach (CPA). They must have a keyworker or care co-ordinator. Implementation of the CPA has been patchy since its introduction in 1991 and there have been several changes in the terminology used. However, it is now fully operational and the CPA remains the foundation of care planning for people with mental health problems who use specialist services. This applies to people who use assertive outreach services too.

The keyworker approach requires one person – the co-ordinator – to take chief responsibility for devising, updating and co-ordinating the treatment and care plan of an individual service user. In addition, the co-ordinator often delivers a great deal of the treatment and care offered. Although arrangements are made to cover leave and other contingencies, it is the co-ordinator who carries specific responsibility for any individual client of the service.

However, one of the key requirements for 'fidelity to the model' of assertive outreach is the use of the team approach. This is quite different from the keyworker approach: the whole team works with all the clients of the service. It is the whole team that considers and agrees the plan and then takes responsibility for work with all clients. This approach was used by those in the USA who first developed assertive community treatment (see above) and has been adopted by some British assertive outreach teams.

The team approach was developed in response to concerns about what would happen if clients became too dependent on one particular staff member. It is an approach that fosters ownership by all staff, and knowledge of and commitment to all clients. It is useful when a worker is unavailable, or when a client and his or her keyworker are having difficulty in working together. It reduces the likelihood of burnout by allowing staff to share responsibility for particularly difficult clients.

However, the team approach does not sit easily with the keyworker approach. British experience has yet to provide a definitive answer on the best way of tackling this aspect of team organisation. Examples of both approaches can be seen across the country. Teams often find a way of taking the best features from each model, meeting the requirements of the CPA while at the same time involving several team members in the care of an individual client.

The Working Together in London teams did initially find it difficult to agree on how best to work. All three fulfilled the requirement to provide a designated care co-ordinator, but they also adopted some aspects of the team approach by agreeing that a small group of workers would relate to particular groups of service users. It may be that in practice 'the distinction between the two approaches is less than is portrayed' (Burns and Firn, 2002).

Summary

- Assertive outreach is a way of organising intensive, user-centred community mental health care and support for people with long-term and serious problems who will not use services.
- Assertive outreach is not a specific treatment in itself, but a vehicle for delivering a range of different treatments and interventions.
- Assertive outreach is a specialist service: it should always be targeted at the people who can derive most benefit from it.
- Assertive outreach derives from the 'assertive community treatment' (ACT) developed in the USA in the 1970s and subsequently adapted for use elsewhere in the world.
- A great deal of research is still going on into assertive outreach, as there is some debate about how far it is transferable from one country to another.
- There is also some difference of opinion about whether there is a list of core criteria that defines 'pure' assertive outreach – and whether absolute fidelity to these criteria is essential for the approach to be effective.
- A team approach is fundamental to assertive outreach, and within the Working Together in London teams there is a debate about the respective merits of this approach and the keyworker approach required by the Care Programme Approach (CPA).

3 Social inclusion and mental health

I never want to go back to the place where I was. I want to be able to cope with the warning signs. Even if there are things happening in the outside world, I want to be able to cope with them. I want to find enjoyment in daily activities.

LEO interviewee

One of the key aims of the Working Together in London programme was to combat the social exclusion experienced by many people with severe and long-term mental health problems. At the time when the programme was being developed, the language of 'exclusion' and 'inclusion' was less familiar in mental health care, but the nature of the problems affecting clients was very well known. Working for inclusion was a critical component of the Working Together in London programme, and indeed the external evaluation concentrates on this aspect.

What is social exclusion?

The terms 'social exclusion' and 'social inclusion' have entered the vocabulary of social policy with surprising rapidity. The Government's Social Exclusion Unit defines exclusion not solely in terms of poverty, but in terms of a group of interconnected factors such as low income, poor housing, low skills and poor education. It is about living on the margins and being cut off from the mainstream.

How does it affect people with mental health problems?

Exclusion works against many groups and individuals in our society, and in many ways. For people who experience mental ill health, there are special factors of discrimination that taken together with other processes create serious problems.

The process of exclusion begins when a person acquires the label 'severely mentally ill'. Society fears mental illness. Nothing will stir up a community more than proposals to bring people with mental health problems into the area, whether they are to live locally or a new hospital or clinic is to be built. The media play their part in exacerbating these prejudices: the desire to sell newspapers or to show more exciting news reports can outweigh any desire to portray a positive image of the people concerned.

As a result, employers, colleagues, landlords, insurers, businesses and others still react negatively to mental illness, and their attitudes stand in the way of a decent quality of life. Despite years of work to combat prejudice, people with mental health problems still experience discrimination. They are often denied the opportunities and rights enjoyed by other members of society, including people with other types of disability.

Fear of the reactions of other people simply adds to the problems experienced by people with serious and long-term mental illness. When they begin to feel unwell, many will isolate themselves from the frightening signs of their illness. But however unpleasant the symptoms may be, the side effects of medication can be just as distressing. It is often said that what the public sees as the symptoms of mental illness are in fact the effects of medication. This was particularly true of the older anti-psychotic medication, and there are many people living in the community who have taken this medication in their time. As a result, those whose appearance and manner are thought to be typical of mentally ill people are often shunned.

What is inclusion?

Inclusion is a positive process of improving rights, access, choice and participation. For people with mental health problems, it is also about access to the best possible treatment and care.

Working for inclusion (Bates, 2002) offers three ways of looking at the subject:

- *Inclusion as access.* An inclusive organisation ensures that all its activities serve the whole community.
- *Inclusion as a decent standard of living.* Everyone, including people with mental health problems, should be able to enjoy a good standard of life, develop their skills and abilities, earn a wage and live in safety in the community.
- *Inclusion as relationships.* Organisations that are inclusive recognise that people need support to develop a network of relationships; these organisations therefore focus upon informal support and community networks.

There are many other ways of looking at inclusion, but they all begin with the vision of a positive process that will enable people to live more fulfilling lives and to play a part in the community.

Working together to bring about inclusion

The Working Together in London programme was designed to bring about inclusion at two levels, the individual and the societal. Assertive outreach teams tackle the whole range of difficulties experienced by their clients. In particular, they are concerned to bring about their inclusion by addressing a wide range of social problems. The Working Together in London teams knew that they would have to address at least the following issues:

Housing

> *I was going to be evicted at one stage, housing benefit was not coming through and I was £1000 in arrears because I was in hospital, and my social worker sorted it out.*
>
> Islington interviewee

People with serious and long-term mental health problems experience difficulty in finding decent housing. They often have little money and cannot easily afford rent or mortgage repayments. If they spend long periods in hospital they may find that they have lost their existing housing – perhaps because the rent or the mortgage has not been paid. Some people who are unwell and do not have good support systems may also be regarded as difficult neighbours and be threatened with eviction.

Employment

I've been thinking about work and getting a job. I'm unemployed at the moment. I worked at a few places but nothing permanent. I was working for a graphic design company. I've been introduced to lots of different people such as an employment officer who works in Hackney and got a CV together but haven't used it yet . . . Can't really commit myself because I don't want to go back to work if it's going to make me ill . . . I need a constructive way of going back into work and not thinking I'm going to be ill.

Islington interviewee

Anyone can lose their job if they are ill for a long period. For people with severe mental health problems, the situation can be exacerbated by the episodic nature of their illness, which often means that they are regarded as unreliable. Prejudice on the part of employers and colleagues can increase the likelihood of job loss. It is also hard to find employment in the first place: even in times of low unemployment, it is the people with serious mental health problems who will have most difficulty in finding work:

We know that disabled people (including those with mental health problems) experience massive disadvantage in the labour market . . . But people with mental health problems are particularly disadvantaged . . . their employment rates are far worse than many other groups of disabled people.

Margaret Hodge, then minister for disabled people at the Department for Education and Employment, quoted in King's Fund, 1999

Education and training

I'm thinking of going back to sixth form college to do GCSE resits, English and Maths. I hope to go to university and do a drama degree . . . I studied a BTEC in health and social care and then went on to psychology, but I was chucked off the course.

Islington interviewee

People with mental health problems may be highly educated, they may have had to drop out of a course in the past, or they may lack even the most basic skills – the range of their potential and their needs is vast. But schools and colleges often know nothing of this: they merely worry that people with mental health problems will be troublesome and require a lot of resources. Colleges have their own priorities about widening participation and raising achievement, and may be concerned that people with mental health problems will push them 'off course' in achieving these objectives. People may therefore find themselves excluded from courses in all but the most basic skills, or may find it difficult to get the support they need even to approach a college.

Financial problems

All in all, I find the experience of being on a low income degrading. I feel I am being punished for being ill and as if it is all my fault, which in turn makes me more depressed.

Respondent to the *Focus on mental health survey*, quoted in Davis and Hill, 2001

People with mental health problems are also disadvantaged by poverty. Because they are often unemployed, they find it hard to bring in a regular income. Life can be precarious for those reliant on benefits. Again, the episodic nature of mental ill health can mean that people recover and want to work again, but fear that if they give up their benefits they will not be able to recover them if health problems recur.

Mental health services

It is important to acknowledge that mental health services themselves have sometimes paid insufficient attention to the whole person. They have tended to concentrate upon symptoms and treatment, neglecting the broader range of difficulties experienced by their clients. When users have had social difficulties, the response of mental health services has often been to refer them on for help but not to deal with the problems directly. Assertive outreach teams are designed to tackle the problems of the 'whole person'.

Mental health services are sometimes guilty of having excessively low expectations of the capacities of their clients. It is often people with the most serious problems who are the subject of this 'poverty of expectation'. By contrast, assertive outreach teams are designed to work with optimism. Although by no means alone in this approach, assertive outreach teams can make a real difference by maintaining high expectations of their clients.

Including all service users

It is important to help individual clients, but it may be equally important to bring about improvements for all users of mental health services. The programme therefore aimed to develop new partnerships that could bring about change at the societal level. The assertive outreach teams would thus offer the opportunity for change at both the individual – team client – level and more broadly for all people with severe and long term mental illness in the area.

The Government endorsed this wider approach in the publication of the *National Service Framework for Mental Health* in 1999. Standard 1 of that Framework requires that:

Health and social services should:
- *Promote mental health for all, working with individuals and communities*
- *Combat discrimination against individuals and groups with mental health problems, and promote their social exclusion.*

Although such thinking was not new, this was the first time it had appeared explicitly in policy guidance. It was further endorsement of the approach taken by the Working Together in London programme.

Working together for local change

The project teams that had led developments in each area were responsible for supporting these partnership initiatives. Work to improve integration within mental health continued: for example, by bringing drug and alcohol services into close working arrangements with assertive outreach. But the broader partnerships were also high on the agenda.

Overall the project teams aimed to make closer contact with:

- housing departments and associations
- adult and continuing education colleges
- employers
- police and probation services
- council services outside the traditional social services department (for example, leisure services)
- welfare benefits agencies
- the wider community.

Chapters 4–6 of this report will say more about the success of the teams in forging new partnerships.

Summary

- One of the key aims of the Working Together in London programme was to combat the social exclusion experienced by many people with severe and long-term mental health problems.
- Exclusion has been described as living on the margins and being cut off from the mainstream.
- For people with severe mental health problems, social exclusion is largely caused by society's ill-informed prejudices about mental illness.
- Social inclusion is a positive process of improving rights, access, choice and participation.
- For the Working Together in London teams, bringing about the social inclusion of people with severe mental health problems meant helping them to solve their difficulties with housing, money, employment, education and training.
- The teams aimed to bring about widespread change in the attitudes of society as a whole, so that not just their clients but everyone with mental health problems in the area would benefit.
- The teams proposed to achieve these changes by making working partnerships with a wide range of other local organisations.

Part two
The three teams

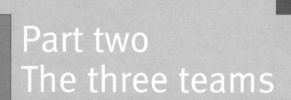

This part of the report describes in detail the three teams that participated in the Working Together in London programme: the Antenna Outreach Service, Haringey; the Islington Assertive Outreach Team; and Lambeth Early Onset (LEO).

In each case, we examine:

- local mental health services before the new team was set up
- the type of service the team offers, and to whom
- the progress the team has made in service integration and in forming partnerships
- the effect it has had on other services
- which of the team's activities have worked well
- which of its activities need improvement
- what the future holds.

Khadija is a young Somalian woman who lives at home with her family. She came to England ten years ago and had difficulties learning English. Shy and timid at school, Khadija left with no formal qualifications. She remained shy and isolated, rarely leaving her home. She didn't want to wash or keep her room clean and she ate very little.

Khadija was referred to mental health services and admitted to hospital under the Mental Health Act, but her family found it difficult to accept that she had a mental health problem. During her hospital stay, Khadija began to communicate with people. She was interested by occupational therapy and was willing to take medication. But, when she went home Khadija's condition gradually worsened again. She refused to take medication or to agree to any treatment.

The assertive outreach team became involved to help Khadija change her behaviour by getting her out into the community and developing a care plan for longer-term development. Staff took her out for short walks and then to local shops and eventually to the cinema. The aim was to help her develop confidence to make informed choices, and to be able to return to education. The team arranged for home tuition and later helped Khadija enrol on a college course.

With intense support from the team's family co-ordinator and from the team psychiatrist, the family has seen the value of medication in helping Khadija to achieve her goals. This has helped her to carry on studying and she now looks after herself better, and keeps her room at home reasonably clean and tidy.

The team will continue to be involved with Khadija to support her in attending her course, and in being a part of the community, as well as maintaining her medication to improve her mental health and her involvement in activities outside the home.

4 The Antenna Outreach Service, Haringey

They care a lot. Sometimes I'm not that realistic and they understand . . . Things are better because of the contact with Antenna. I know who I am now. They care for me and care about me.

Antenna interviewee

I'm talking more, not bottling up problems. It's someone to talk to, and I got the flat out of them.

Antenna interviewee

Meeting the needs of young black people was the top priority for the Antenna Outreach Service in Haringey. There were very high rates of mental illness locally, and a disproportionate number of black people were affected. Although a fairly well developed range of community mental health services existed, they did not adequately serve younger people from the African and Caribbean communities. A new approach was needed to fill this gap. Therefore a broad consortium of organisations – including health and social care commissioners and providers (including Haringey Healthcare NHS Trust and local government), mental health groups, housing agencies, education drop-in services and the local black African and black African-Caribbean communities – developed a bid to participate in the Working Together in London programme.

The proposed service would concentrate on people aged 16 to 25 who had already experienced the onset of a serious mental health problem. The aim was to work assertively to establish contact and to offer treatment, care and support. The local black communities had some suspicions of mental health services, fearing that the only options available for their young people were medication or a hospital bed. The new team owed its existence to these concerns, and it addressed them directly by providing a focused service. The team also aimed to offer advice and support to the families and carers of the young people, working to keep families and support networks together.

The team would offer a culturally sensitive service, using workers recruited from the African and Caribbean communities. It would also concentrate on working within youth culture. Young people experiencing the onset of serious mental health problems are in all other respects no different from their peers. They want the same things – friendships, good education, a job, music, clothes and places to go – and therefore they are particularly reluctant to acquire the label 'mental illness'. To enable the team to draw upon the experience of young people locally, a peer support group – the Antenna Group – was set up.

Addressing the needs of younger black people with mental health problems would take the team beyond the boundaries of mental health care. To be effective, it needed to work in an integrated way with other services – but it also needed to form partnerships with agencies outside the usual mental health network. In accordance with the interests of the young people themselves, the team targeted agencies in the fields of education, training, employment and leisure services.

The Antenna project was ambitious and set itself taxing targets. It was working with a group of clients new to the service, and the communities involved had high expectations.

Criteria for acceptance by Antenna

- African/African Caribbean
- Aged 16–25
- No more than two hospital admissions
- Suffering from mental illness
- Lives in Tottenham or Edmonton (the team does not serve the whole of Haringey)

What were existing mental health services like in Haringey?

Before Antenna was set up, mental health services in the area were mainly provided by Haringey Healthcare NHS Trust, which covered the London Borough of Haringey as well as the Edmonton area of the London Borough of Enfield. The combined population in 1998 was 300,980. The area has an average MINI score of 112.9.* In April 2001 a larger mental health trust was formed, taking responsibility for Barnet, Enfield and Haringey. However, in order to provide consistent information on how the assertive outreach team functioned, this chapter concentrates on the area covered by the earlier trust.

In Haringey and Edmonton (hereafter referred to as 'Haringey' for convenience), St Ann's Hospital provides most of the in-patient care. There is also a 'ward in the community' for people requiring rehabilitation in an in-patient setting. the trust also has medium secure forensic beds in Camlet Lodge at Chase Farm Hospital, Enfield.

The community mental health teams (CMHTs) in Haringey are multidisciplinary, with social services and health care input. There are five sectors (Edmonton, Wood Green, Tottenham, Hornsey and Highgate), each with one CMHT. In addition, there is a social services community support team, TULIP – a voluntary sector mental health provider – a dual diagnosis team and Antenna. Details of service provision are given in Table 1.

---

* **MINI index** An index for small areas that uses the characteristics of the local population (as measured in the 1991 census) to predict the distribution of need for mental health services. Specifically, it looks at the indicators of social isolation (married, single, divorced), poverty (car/no car), unemployment, permanent sickness and temporary and insecure housing tenure. For example, areas where a high percentage of the population is single, widowed or divorced and lives in temporary and insecure housing are predicted to have greater needs for mental health services than areas where the population demonstrates a lower prevalence of these characteristics. The higher the index number, the greater the need.

Table 1: The provision of mental health services across Haringey		
Service	Total provision	Provision per 100K population
In-patient beds		
Acute	130	63
ICU	12	6
Forensic	16	8
Rehabilitation	46	22
Total	204	98
Residential care places	256	166
Day care units	10	4.8
Mental health teams	9	4.3
Note: figures were supplied in 2001 and have been updated, where possible, in 2002.		

What kind of service?

The local steering group was committed to:

- *providing culturally specific emotional support and care* by encouraging the use of a range of approaches to mental health management – not only within the new assertive outreach team but also within mainstream services
- *linking with, and using, wider community networks* and organisations where young people congregate: for example, cultural centres, youth clubs, music centres, libraries and church premises
- *using a range of clinical interventions*, including short-term problem-solving approaches, family interventions and/or support, medication, identification of indicators of relapse and crisis planning for the future
- *engaging assertively with other care and support services* to prevent, as far as possible, compulsory admission to hospital
- *facilitating early discharge* through continuing contact with clients and maintaining their accommodation and community support systems
- *providing continuing assertive support and treatment* using the range of expertise in the team
- *acting as a single point of contact for all aspects of care and support*, thus reducing the need for users to contact several different services, which can act as a deterrent.

Antenna was designed to operate 365 days of the year and to be able to provide a response outside normal office hours. It was clear from the beginning that the service planned to stick with its clients over the long term. The principle it followed in all its work was 'first in and last out'.

The service was formally launched in July 1999, at a local church much used by African and African-Caribbean people. Over 100 people attended.

Table 2: The composition and operational details of the Antenna team 1999	
Date became operational	October 1999
Number of staff	10
Staff composition	1 team leader 1 project manager 1 consultant psychiatrist 1 social worker 3 outreach workers 1 admin co-ordinator 1 family support co-ordinator (P/T) 1 occupational technician (P/T)
Caseload	50
Staff to client ratio	1:6
Upper staff to client limit	1:10
Upper caseload limit	50
Main hours of operation	9am–5pm Mon–Fri, 4 hours Sat–Sun
Out of hours	24 hour on-call via mobile phone

In 2001–2 the staff costs of Antenna amounted to £259,000 and the fixed and running costs to a further £46,500, giving a total of £305,500. With the then caseload of around 50, this meant that the cost per client per year was about £6100.

The Antenna Youth Group

The steering group specifically sought the support of young people. A group of individuals who reflected the wider youth community were therefore invited to participate. Their task was to help shape the new service with their ideas and to share their experiences of youth culture and current trends. They would also help with recruiting some of the team members. The steering group recruited young people who had used mental health services, had experience of youth work or mental health, or had had contact with:

- general youth services, statutory and voluntary
- church youth groups
- education and employment
- Leaving Care team
- youth cultural groups.

The young people were told that their involvement would bring them reciprocal benefits, including:

- experience in developing a new public service
- experience of selecting staff
- committee and presentation skills
- opportunity to make local services better.

The youth group also developed distinctive client information and marketing material for the whole service. In essence, the working ethos of the Antenna Youth Group was 'hearing and respecting the views of others'.

The first year

Antenna had some initial recruitment problems: for instance, it had difficulty in finding a black approved social worker through the links with the local authority. The team thought it might opt for recruiting a black social worker and offering special training in mental health. In the event, the NHS trust arranged a secondment and the matter was resolved, but relationships with Haringey Social Services were strained by the incident.

There was also some difficulty at first in finding a consultant psychiatrist from the same ethnic group as the team, but this appointment was successfully made later in the first year. Three black outreach workers were recruited who had good experience in working with young people with mental health problems. The team also included a black occupational therapist, whose role would primarily be to help young black people improve their life skills – particularly important after discharge from hospital. The family support worker was a part-time post to support the needs of carers, including liaison with the Haringey carers' organisation; the team felt that this was a function often overlooked by mental health services.

> *I live with grandparents . . . My family are more understanding now that they [Antenna] came round. Family can socialise now . . . Every time I mention my friend that was stabbed and died my grandparents go ape, but I want Antenna to explain to them that I'm still hurting.*

Antenna interviewee

The services found new premises in Tottenham, and the first five days of SCMH training were successfully completed.

As planned, Antenna recruited its clients gradually over the first year. At this early stage the team leader spent a great deal of time talking to the community mental health teams and to a range of other agencies. The team assessed clients from these agencies as well as from the CMHTs.

Progress in service integration

The team not only worked closely with the CMHTs, but also formed links with the dual diagnosis service. Many clients were using drugs and alcohol as well as suffering from mental health problems. Antenna and the dual diagnosis service worked well together and helped a number of clients, many of whom were jointly assessed at a time of crisis. Psychiatrists in other mental health teams soon began to refer their clients to Antenna. Integration with other mental health services increased during the first year.

One of the aims of Antenna had been to work closely with general practitioners. However, this has proved difficult: considerable effort was made during the first year to discuss the service with GPs, but only a few referred potential clients. This low level of contact has persisted. However, direct contact with certain GPs was good and the then primary care groups were helpful. It may be that the clients of

Antenna had been too remote from primary care services, and did not regard themselves as having a health problem. Also, GPs may not have recognised the opportunity for early intervention in mental health problems.

Progress in partnerships

Antenna formed successful partnerships with a number of agencies: for example, the borough's leisure services, which subsidised the cost of hiring a hall and a coach for the weekly sports group. In return, the team gave basic education in mental health issues to borough youth workers – an important contribution towards the social inclusion of young people with mental health problems.

> *With the sports group we would have talking sessions first, about the things going round in our heads. Then play football or do some weights.*
>
> Antenna interviewee

The team also formed working relationships with the youth and education services. Clients successfully completed the Prince's Youth Trust twelve-week work experience programme run by education and youth services. The team also worked with local employment agencies, and in the first year five clients joined courses at the local adult and continuing education college.

> *I go to college. I'm retaking GCSEs . . . I took care of organising this myself.*
>
> Antenna interviewee

A major problem was arranging accommodation for clients. Housing people with mental health problems is known to be difficult and Antenna's experience has borne this out. Clients aged between 16 and 17 are unable to sign tenancy agreements, and very young people are difficult to support in independent housing.

> *I live round this area in a one bedroom flat. Antenna helped me to get that. I moved in a month ago. I had been living in a group home for a year.*
>
> Antenna interviewee

The team has worked closely with organisations from the black community, including the Pyramid counselling service, Inspire Dance Company, Nehandea Black women's group and others. Links were formed with the churches and have remained strong throughout the programme. Antenna has also worked with others engaged in promoting black mental health: for example, with the Sainsbury Centre for Mental Health on the Breaking the Circles of Fear programme (Sainsbury Centre for Mental Health, 2002).

> *I feel that because they are black they understand more about being a black girl.*
>
> Antenna interviewee

> *It's nice to know there is just an Afro-Caribbean service, but I also like to mix with others.*
>
> Antenna interviewee

The second year

Antenna grew from strength to strength in its second year:

- 57 clients had been fully assessed.
- 47 clients were 'on the books', and the other ten clients assessed had been referred to other services with support from Antenna.
- Antenna's helpline received 220 calls.

The support for carers was widely welcomed in the local community, where carers had previously felt cut off from mental health services. Core staff remained in post, although there were some vacancies. Problems over the approved social worker persisted: because of the secondment arrangement, the borough was not prepared to offer supervision and support. However, working relationships continued at the team-to-team level.

Progress in service integration

Antenna continued to develop its links with other mental health services – primarily the CMHTs, the dual diagnosis team and the child and adolescent mental health services.

Progress in partnerships

The team further developed its partnerships with the borough sports and leisure section, leading to the expansion of the sports and leisure programme for clients.

> *We go bowling, do different activities. We do it as a big group. We went on a weekend break to Brighton.*
>
> Antenna interviewee

Good links were maintained with the youth and education services, which benefited individual clients and raised general awareness of the needs of young people with mental health problems.

The Antenna Youth Group continued to provide strong support. It helped to develop service information, and also promoted a video. Produced in 2000, the video *Heavy Mental* deals with mental health in urban communities. It aims to remove the 'heavy stones of ignorance' about mental illness and mental health. The video was highly successful and has been used in youth work throughout the borough. *Heavy Mental* received its first showing at an evening of entertainment held in the local black community centre. Over 300 people attended to see the video and to listen to music and poetry, all of it devoted to the theme of improving mental health. Many of the contributors had been users of mental health services at some time in their lives.

Effects on other services

Use of hospital beds has gone up in Haringey, but it is not possible to be clear about why this is so and how far it is attributable to Antenna. Assertive outreach services may reduce the use of hospital beds over a period of time longer than the life of this study. They can reduce the necessity for compulsory admissions by enabling careful monitoring of the condition of specific clients, and can decrease lengths of stay by improving discharge plans and practice. Working Together in London was too short a programme to offer significant evidence on this point.

Trends such as an increase in bed use are bound to affect decisions by funders on whether to continue to support an innovative community service of this kind. However, Haringey managers have said that Antenna's funding is secure.

What has worked well

Antenna itself and local stakeholders and service users have broadly agreed on what have been the most successful aspects of the service to date:

- its use of a psycho-social model of care, which has provided acceptable and effective treatment, care and support
- the family/parent support service, which has provided effective psycho-education
- the telephone referral system, which has saved time and paperwork
- the 24-hour helpline
- the team approach, which has enabled the team to function well and retain staff
- the engagement with the wider community, which has developed very successfully (this includes not only statutory agencies outside the NHS but also the local voluntary sector and community groups)
- the Antenna Youth Group, which has helped the team and its clients to keep in touch with youth culture, and whose members have acted as ambassadors and educators in the local community.

What needs improvement

> *Even though they were nice people, they did make the situation worse. They didn't know how to deal with the family. They didn't know how to deal with the situation. They would say that Mum shouldn't do and say certain things . . . Things changed for the better, but not because they really helped. In a way they did help, but they could have done it better. Maybe it's a training matter. They identified the problems and then I solved them . . . The people were nice but they didn't really deal with the situation.*
>
> Antenna interviewee

The team itself identified the following issues as needing further development. They pose a challenge to all mental health services in urban areas:

- acquiring an understanding of how services can best respond to cultural issues in relation to both black services and youth services
- bringing an understanding of culturally specific approaches into mainstream mental health services
- improving integration between functional services (such as assertive outreach) and more generalist services (such as community mental health teams)
- advising commissioners about new functional services and the benefits they bring to specific groups of mental health users.

The future

I think that they need to get more staff.

Antenna interviewee

I would get more young people involved.

Antenna interviewee

Antenna looks forward to continuing growth within Haringey's mental health services. In particular, by:

- expanding from Tottenham and Edmonton to cover other areas of Haringey
- building on the psycho-social model in partnership with other services
- building upon its links with the community
- building upon its links with services outside mental health in order to increase their capacity to help people with mental health problems.

5 The Islington Assertive Outreach Team

It's like having a bigger brother . . . The AO team are brilliant . . . The AO team has been very supportive. Everything is just on an even keel . . . Compared to previous community care team the AO team is much less formal . . . They always phone up to see how you are and not just on an appointment day.

Islington interviewee

I have a great relationship with the social worker. I feel we can talk and he helps me fill out forms. He knows me quite well, we've been together for the last two years . . . They're a bloody good crowd . . .I can talk to the team about anything.

Islington interviewee

The Islington assertive outreach team focuses on people aged 18 to 65 who have severe mental health problems. Based at a large primary care practice, it works closely with the local crisis team and community mental health teams. Links with local communities – especially black and minority ethnic groups and the voluntary sector – are a major priority for the team.

Islington and its neighbour Camden have very high rates of mental illness. Although there was a wide range of services at the time of this study, the connections between them were not always clear. The decision was therefore taken to remodel the mental health and social care services completely. A new assertive outreach service would meet the need for targeted community support for people with serious mental health problems. This was at least partly a response to a series of local tragedies, where people with severe problems had remained in the community with little support and went on to harm other people. It was also hoped that the new service would reduce the demand for hospital beds by providing a more appropriate response.

The assertive outreach team for South Islington was to form the basis of the new service and would provide a model for later developments in North Islington and Camden. The new service would also work to improve service integration, in order to avoid yet further fragmentation of mental health care in a locality where many teams and services existed but integration was said to be poor.

A consortium of health and social care commissioners and providers had worked with the strong local user groups and the voluntary sector to agree on the key local problems. They had identified a significant group of people with serious and long-term mental health problems who did not willingly engage with existing services – although they were frequent users of in-patient beds, usually compulsorily. Many had parallel problems of substance misuse and they experienced difficulties with housing, welfare benefits and isolation. The consortium's aim was to develop an assertive outreach team to engage with, treat and support this group of people.

Islington has a multi-racial community with a wide variety of ethnic groups represented. It also has a large number of voluntary and community groups. The new service therefore needed to address the needs of people from a range of ethnically diverse groups and to do this in collaboration with the statutory and voluntary agencies of the area. This challenge could only be met by improving service integration and broader inter-agency partnerships.

A randomised controlled trial (RCT) of the team was also carried out.

Criteria for acceptance by the Islington Assertive Outreach Team

- Aged 18–65
- A severe and enduring mental illness
- Known to statutory and voluntary agencies for at least 12 months
- History of poor engagement
- One admission of 50 days or more in the past year or one admission of over 100 days in the past 12–24 months or three admissions in the past 12 months or five admissions in the past two years
- No severe personality disorder, primary substance misuse or organic disorder.

What were existing mental health services like in Islington?

The London Borough of Islington has around 179,000 people, of whom an estimated 123,510 are aged between 15 and 64. Islington's MINI score of 122.4 means that it has the highest level of mental health needs in the capital.

Camden and Islington Mental Health NHS Trust provided mental health services at the time when this review was carried out (it is now the Camden and Islington Mental Health and Social Care Trust, but this does not affect our findings). In-patient care in Islington is mostly provided by the Waterlow Unit in Highgate, near the local acute general hospital; some beds are also available further north at St Luke's Hospital, which is in a neighbouring borough. Like Haringey, Islington uses the medium secure forensic beds at Camlet Lodge. There is a women's crisis house at Drayton Park, which serves as an alternative for women to acute in-patient care.

Residential care was provided by the NHS trust, the social services department and a number of independent sector organisations. Much of this residential care was set up in the wake of the closure of Friern Hospital in 1993. An accommodation review has led to major changes in provision, as it was found that there was an oversupply of 24-hour staffed units and a scarcity of less intensively staffed units. The nature of this accommodation is critical in view of the requirements of people with serious and long-term mental health problems. Most of them will never have been in one of the old Victorian asylums and they will aspire to very different housing solutions.

Islington has multi-disciplinary teams operating from five community mental health centres (Calshot, Canonbury, Elthorne, Drayton and Archway.) A crisis

Table 3: The provision of mental health services across Islington

Service	Total provision	Provision per 100K population
In-patient beds		
Acute	72	59
ICU	7	6
Forensic	21	17
Rehabilitation	26	21
Total	126	103
Residential care places	384	311
Day care units	7	5.7
Mental health teams	7	5.7

Note: figures were supplied in 2001 and have been updated, where possible, in 2002.

resolution team, which treats people with acute mental health problems in their homes, also operates in Islington alongside the assertive outreach team. Table 3 gives details of the service provision across Islington.

What kind of service?

The South Islington Team was set up as part of the reorganised mental health strategy for Camden and Islington. The new approach involved dividing the area into four quadrants, with South Islington in the south-east corner. Each quadrant was to include a community mental health team (CMHT), working in liaison with primary care. Each team was to be linked to in-patient beds and to the new crisis resolution teams working in the community to keep people out of hospital. The assertive outreach teams were to offer an innovative way of working with people who have serious and long-term mental health problems.

The assertive outreach service concentrated on integration with other mental health services, including:

- CMHTs
- crisis resolution team
- day services
- primary care groups
- drug and alcohol services
- forensic services.

The input of users and the local carers group was critical to the development of the service, and these links had to be maintained. Indeed, some of the funding was used to improve user training for the wider Camden and Islington service.

The new team also set out to improve partnerships with organisations outside mental health. At the outset, the following organisations were thought to be the most important:

- housing and the housing support team
- welfare rights and in particular the specialist Islington welfare rights service
- employment projects in the area
- centres and groups working with people from black and minority ethnic communities.

It was always expected that, in addition to experiencing mental health problems, many clients of the South Islington team would be using illicit drugs and alcohol. As one of its early goals, the team set out to acquire expertise in working with this type of client.

The annual cost of the team was around £364,000. With the then caseload of 66, this meant a cost of £5,515 per client per year.

Table 4: The composition and operational details of the Islington Assertive Outreach Team 1999	
Date became operational	November 1999
Number of staff	11
Staff composition	1 team leader (H Grade nurse) 1 deputy team leader (senior social worker) 1 consultant (half-time) 3 psychiatric nurses (G Grade) 1 social worker 1 occupational therapist 1 clinical psychologist (half-time) 2 support workers
Caseload	66
Staff to client ratio	1:7
Upper staff to client limit	1:10
Upper caseload limit	95
Main hours of operation	9am–8pm Mon–Fri, 10am–6pm Sat–Sun
Out of hours	No on-call arrangements within AO team itself, but links with local crisis team

The research programme

The South Islington team was to be the subject not only of evaluation as part of the Working Together in London programme but also of a randomised controlled trial (RCT) of the assertive outreach intervention. Chapter 9 reports on the evaluation of the Working Together in London programme. The RCT is not covered in this study, but will be reported separately; at the time of writing, the findings are expected to appear late in 2004.

The RCT was designed to:

1. Assess the clinical and cost effectiveness of the assertive outreach team.
2. Assess whether the team faithfully implements assertive outreach, taking into consideration:
   - the validity of the benefits reported in the international literature
   - the effectiveness, in terms of personal health and social adaptation, for patients receiving such care.

The first year

The team was generally able to recruit the staff it wanted – even at a time of major changes in services, when people can be reluctant to move. There was, however, a problem over recruitment for the support worker post. This was designed as a job share for two service users yet, despite attempts to recruit through a range of media, it was not filled. The team felt that the salary offered might have been insufficient to persuade people to take the huge step of coming off welfare benefits.

In view of the reorganisation of services in Camden and Islington, it was perhaps inevitable that integrated working should be difficult to begin with. The CMHTs were unsure of the role of the new team. This led them to refer some existing clients who were unsuitable for assertive outreach, and to fail to refer others who might have been helped.

The team also believed that the RCT created some initial difficulties. As part of the research project, some clients who had been referred for assertive outreach services and were thought to be suitable were referred back for 'ordinary' care, usually the community mental health services. The research was known to be important for establishing the effectiveness of the team, but the processes involved in it were thought to have caused some early difficulties in integration between teams.

By the end of the first full year of operation, the team had:

- 49 clients 'on the books'; 100 people had been referred for assessment and allocated either to the team or to 'ordinary' care, and a further 20 were under consideration as to their suitability
- a full complement of staff, but there were emerging concerns about turnover.

The high staff turnover arose from the fact that team members felt under considerable pressure because of the weight and complexity of the problems experienced by clients. This problem has persisted.

Progress in service integration

Collaboration with other mental health services improved during the first year. Contacts with primary care were limited, but this was thought to be because many of the clients had been out of touch with mainstream services for years and had only experienced specialist mental health care – often compulsorily. Links with primary care are still limited to the few clients who do visit a GP. Contact had, however, been made with the then primary care groups.

Progress in partnerships

For the South Islington team, housing has proved an enduring problem. The London Borough of Islington Housing Department was being reorganised when the team was first set up, so it was not easy to make the right links. The team's clients had often had major housing problems in the past. They were not easy people to deal with: some had been unable to pay the rent, others had been difficult neighbours. In fact, housing was the key social problem for some clients.

Links with black and minority ethnic communities progressed slowly at first. However, good working relationships were developed with the Lambo Centre, where black clients were able to participate in social activities.

> I don't see many black people working in the AO team. I haven't seen any black members. I prefer to have white workers, but for others it might be good and to have more of a balance.

Islington interviewee

The second year

By the end of the team's second year of operation, integration and partnership working had continued to develop satisfactorily.

> I work here [at the clubhouse] four and a half days a week and work elsewhere [in a library earning £15 a week] two and a half days a week . . . I'm doing voluntary work to see if I like doing it before jumping into a full-time job . . . I could easily be back at work but I need to be working off my own motivation to get things done.

Islington interviewee

Progress in partnerships

Two new workers joined the team to help develop its work with black and minority ethnic (BME) groups. Recruited through a collaboration with KUSH, a black-led housing and mental health organisation, the new workers had helped clients to make contact with BME community organisations and services.

The problems of finding appropriate accommodation for clients, and then of helping them to remain housed, have persisted. The borough housing service created a new accommodation team to help tackle these issues by improving joint working on particular cases. Umbrella, a mental health charity, has also been helpful in this matter.

> They've organised my housing, which was my main area of concern. I went into hospital and then went to a rehabilitation home and then they found me a flat.

Islington interviewee

Staff turnover was still a problem. The team manager thought it might be connected with burnout. Team working had not been as effective as hoped – some staff accepted the approach, others wanted to use the keyworker approach – and this may have contributed to the problem.

One particularly challenging group of clients were those with very complex benefits problems, and the team felt it needed more specialist support to work with them.

> *They help with benefits, to fill out forms and back up statements.*
> Islington interviewee

Working with dual diagnosis

An early aim of the team was to find new ways of working with clients who had a dual diagnosis of mental health problems and substance misuse. In 2000 a group of workers from Camden and Islington visited the service in New Hampshire, USA, which has an international reputation for assertive community treatment for clients with a dual diagnosis. Two members of the Islington Assertive Outreach team were part of the group and were subsequently able to develop new ways of working within the team. They also joined an in-house group offering training to all the mental health teams in Camden and Islington.

Policy developments have reinforced the importance of this training. In its recent publication *Mental health policy guide: dual diagnosis good practice guide* (Department of Health, 2002), the Department of Health emphasises that all staff of assertive outreach teams must be trained to deal with dual diagnosis.

Effects on other services

The team has drawn its caseload largely from the CMHTs in the area, but there is no evidence that any other 'substitution effects' have taken place. As in Haringey, there has been some increase in in-patient care – but also as in Haringey, it is difficult to establish the cause. At any time there are around 10 clients of the assertive team on in-patient wards, and it is felt that about six of these clients require long-term 24-hour care. This suggests that they are inappropriate clients for the team, and that greater clarity is needed about which clients are best served by assertive outreach. It may also suggest that, while the team can improve its operation, any reduction in the use of beds will only be observable over a longer time scale.

The crisis resolution team is seen as the main way to reduce bed usage, providing an appropriate substitute service and releasing resources.

The introduction of the assertive outreach service was expected to give the CMHTs more time to devote to other clients. But this has not happened: any spare capacity has been filled, and it seems that need has not levelled off but increased. The CMHTs are the same size as before, but the introduction of assertive outreach has at least enabled them to work more with primary care, so meeting one of Islington's aims when setting up the new service.

What has worked well

The team and local stakeholders have identified the following areas where they feel progress was made in the operation of the assertive outreach team during the first two years:

- the introduction of daily handover/planning meetings
- a 'medication run' to reach clients who present daily problems
- the use of a 'crisis board'
- the recruitment of a specialist housing and benefits worker into the team
- the introduction of regular team sessions with the consultant for substance misuse.

What needs improvement

However, there are other areas where further improvement is felt to be needed.

> *I've been seeing them since December. The team before was better. They kept their appointments and didn't allow time to drift. It was easier to get used to one person but now I have three or four . . . I wouldn't like to wait so long between seeing them. Because of their workload I have to see more than one person but they're busy, so I see them every three or four weeks . . . I would prefer two to three weeks. I get on very well with the workers . . . I haven't told them that I would like to see them more . . . I wouldn't say life has changed, because I haven't had much contact, so I don't yet know what they are capable of doing with me.*
>
> Islington interviewee

The caseload of the team was originally intended to be 90, but this has proved impossible to achieve. Some members of the team think that even the current workload of 66 is too high. Assertive outreach teams are not set up to achieve a specific throughput, and this may lead some team members to feel that they are being overworked as more new clients join the team. Benefits and accommodation work take up a lot of staff time, and there are moves to enable the team to function more effectively.

Local managers have suggested that three types of people currently being seen by the team are inappropriate as clients:

- people with whom the team has achieved some success: for example, those who now require one visit per week, have a care plan and can be discharged to the CMHT
- people using the hospital long term, for whom another kind of residential service may be required
- people for whom assertive outreach is not adding value and where no change is expected; they too could perhaps be discharged back to the CMHT.

Links have been initiated between the team and agencies in the community, but there is still some way to go before these links can materially help the South Islington clients, who have long histories of severe mental ill health and experience serious social exclusion. What may be emerging is a team that is learning how best to work with clients who have some of the most complex and longstanding problems in mental health care. The wider task of achieving greater social inclusion is proceeding more slowly.

The future

It's a pity they haven't got bigger offices.

Islington interviewee

How will the Islington team be funded in future? Fortunately, mental health services have received top-level support from the Camden and Islington Health Authority, which has provided extra investment that should cover the cost of the team. Additional resources have been made available through the accommodation review. Money has also been received for employment services, which will pay for an employment co-ordinator to join the assertive outreach team. Future decisions will also reflect the findings of the randomised controlled trial: two assertive outreach teams may be developed – one for North Islington as well as one for South Islington.

For their part, the South Islington team and the local steering group both believe that there is a positive future for assertive outreach. However, a number of important issues remain to be tackled:

■ A realistic appreciation is needed of the severe difficulties experienced by clients and of the time required to address them (a reduction in, for example, the use of in-patient beds will clearly take time).
■ The approach to team working needs to be strengthened.
■ Links with the crisis resolution teams need to be improved, to ensure that clients receive the most appropriate community-based service.
■ Certain team processes require improvement: for example, there is a need for standardised assessments, cross-professional training, a standard set of criteria for client discharge and transfer across Islington, and a more flexible approach to working hours.
■ Accessible material should be developed for clients and carers on the operation of assertive outreach and other teams in the new system.
■ Further work is needed with community organisations, building on the work led by KUSH and on the plans for a lunch club and sports group.

6 Lambeth Early Onset (LEO)

LEO have brought me a better understanding of mental illness and I feel able to deal with it. Before I ignored it and I wasn't able to deal with it and I didn't want to accept help.

LEO interviewee

LEO have made it known that it's just a blip . . . LEO being so open and positive has helped.

LEO interviewee

Lambeth Early Onset (LEO) is an assertive outreach service that focuses on young people aged from 16 to 30, placing special emphasis on psycho-social interventions. The team has links with a broad range of agencies in the voluntary sector (especially the BME voluntary sector), primary care and criminal justice. Other partnerships are connected with education, training and employment, and the team is also linked to the local Health Action Zone (HAZ).

Plans for the new service were developed by a consortium of organisations, including mental health, primary care and housing agencies, voluntary groups from the black community, the Lambeth HAZ, the police and the probation service. The consortium had identified a need for better services for younger people who had developed serious mental health problems.

The Lambeth HAZ had itself focused on young people across the borough, with an emphasis on education, training and employment as well as on access to health care. This provided an ideal opportunity for mental health services to play their part too. They could work with a broad range of agencies already active in the area to bring about the social inclusion of young people with health and other problems.

The NHS had a particular interest in developing an assertive outreach team to offer treatment, care and support to people who would not voluntarily use mental health services. The aim was to target those who were experiencing the onset of serious mental illness but whose age and interests led them to avoid anything that might label them as 'having mental illness'. The team would work to reduce the trauma of early contacts with mental health services and to promote the recovery and social integration of the clients. There was to be a special emphasis on offering information and support to carers and families, with the aim of keeping younger people in contact with their support networks.

Lambeth had already set up a wide range of mental health services, so the new team would also need to promote closer integration in order to avoid duplication of effort and fragmentation of the 'net of care'.

This ambitious project also aimed to foster positive community responses and to play its part in improving the health of the community, working to develop education, training and work opportunities.

Criteria for acceptance by the LEO team

- First or second episode of psychosis
- Aged 16–40
- Lives in borough of Lambeth
- No primary diagnosis of drug or alcohol disorder
- Does not have an existing keyworker within a CMHT

What were existing mental health services like in Lambeth?

With around 269,500 people – including 185,955 between the ages of 15 and 64 – Lambeth is the fifth most heavily populated borough in the capital and the most heavily populated of the inner London boroughs. Lambeth has a MINI score of 119.9, the fifth highest in London. Mental health services are provided by the South London and Maudsley NHS Trust.

In-patient care for Lambeth is based at the Maudsley Hospital, Lambeth Hospital and St Thomas's Hospital. The borough's medium secure forensic beds are at the Caine Hill Unit in Coulsdon, Surrey. Lambeth has only recently set up integrated health and social services community teams in its five sectors. In four of the sectors (North, South West, North East and North West), there are two teams – an assessment and treatment team and a case management team. In the South East sector there is a single community team. There are also the following borough-wide services: a community rehabilitation team, a community forensic team and

Table 5: The provision of mental health services across Lambeth		
Service	**Total provision**	**Provision per 100K population**
In-patient beds		
Acute	116	62
ICU	16.7	10
Forensic	118	63
Rehabilitation	43	23
Total	293.7	160
Residential care places	216	116
Day care units	8	4.3
Mental health teams	14	8
Note: figures were supplied in 2001 and have been updated, where possible, in 2002.		

the Lambeth Early Onset (LEO) team. The trust and Lambeth social services department provide day care and, as in the other Working Together in London areas, the trust, social services and the independent sector between them provide residential care. The extent of service provision is described in Table 5.

What kind of service?

LEO aims to improve clinical and social outcomes for clients by:

- early identification of their problems
- assessment of their needs for treatment, care and support
- treatment of mental health problems
- offering family, vocational and educational support to carers.

The service started life as Lambeth Early Intervention Service but was soon renamed Lambeth Early Onset (LEO).

LEO was designed to meet the need for outreach, safe and secure in-patient care and a range of activities; the whole service is able to respond 365 days of the year and out of normal office hours. Developed as part of a much broader service that would work with younger and more vulnerable people, it was to include a small number of dedicated in-patient beds in a new unit at Lambeth Hospital.

During the initial stages of a person's illness, their vital links with family, relatives and social networks are usually still intact. If there is early intervention, these networks can perhaps be preserved. LEO would work assertively to strengthen and

Table 6: The composition and operational details of the LEO team 2000	
Date became operational	January 2000
Number of staff	13
Staff composition	1 team leader (acting) 1 consultant 1 specialist registrar 1 social worker 1 development worker 2 nurses (G Grade) 2 nurses (G Grade) 1 psychologist 2 health care assistants 1 administrator
Caseload	60
Staff to client ratio	1:5
Upper staff to client limit	1:15
Upper caseload limit	90
Main hours of operation	8am–8pm Mon–Fri, 9am–5pm Sat–Sun
Out of hours	24 hour on-call via mobile phone

extend these links and to re-establish those that had already broken down. This way of working aimed to prevent the breakdown in contact that leads to loneliness and isolation for many people with long-term mental illness.

Improving working relationships and partnerships were particularly important aims for LEO. The reorganisation of services was posing a considerable challenge to the staff of all community mental health teams. The new team would need to play its part in bringing about more effective integration within the mental health system. Wider partnership working was equally important if LEO was to maintain contact with other initiatives for young people. It was therefore regarded as important for the team to include a dedicated development worker who did not have a client caseload.

The annual cost of the LEO community team was £322,025 and the caseload was around 60. This gives a figure of £5367 per client per year.

The research programme

LEO was also to be the subject of a randomised controlled trial (RCT) to look at the effectiveness of the assertive outreach team. As with Islington, the findings of the trial will not be reported here, but will be published late in 2003.

The first year

At the time when LEO was being set up, the scale of local reorganisation created some difficulties for the new team. A new NHS mental health trust was coming into being, and with all staff having to compete for their posts in the trust, there was uncertainty about the wisdom of joining a new service. Recruitment began in 1999, but the full staff complement was not achieved until early 2000. The team itself got off to a slow start, but functioned well later.

Work began in January 2000, and the team took on clients slowly at first to avoid overload. These clients were incorporated into the RCT.

The training package offered by the SCMH was particularly helpful. Team members were already skilled in many aspects of the work they were to undertake, but the team leader commented at the time on the importance of the whole team training together. Interestingly, the team specifically requested training in dual diagnosis interventions even at that early stage.

Progress in service integration

Collaboration with other mental health teams progressed satisfactorily. The clients allocated to LEO responded well and seemed willing to engage with the new service. Links were established with child and adolescent mental health services (CAMHs). This link became particularly important for clients who had young children of their own, as the CAMHs were able to help the team deal with the difficulties experienced by children whose parents have mental health problems.

Although the team did manage to contact individual general practitioners, and the then PCG was a member of the consortium supporting the project, links with GPs were on the whole disappointing. The requirements of the research study exacerbated the problem: if an individual was appropriately referred, but was then returned for 'ordinary' care, GPs in the area might lose confidence in the new service. The team therefore concentrated on making broader links with primary care early on.

Progress in partnerships

The development worker began by contacting, and sometimes visiting, organisations concerned with young people and with black and minority ethnic communities. In the first six months, she made contact with:

- Lambeth College, to raise awareness of mental health across the college (not just to staff working with students with special needs)
- local schools, to raise awareness of the importance of good mental health and to combat stigma (this work was part of a broader community education programme linked to the HAZ)
- voluntary groups that had helped to support the team.

The second year

They put me in touch with solicitors, insurers and the local authority. I had problems with mortgage arrears and they patched me through to the solicitors.

LEO interviewee

A year after it started work, the LEO team had 41 clients. A further 41 people had been assessed but referred for other services as part of the RCT.

The in-patient unit opened in March 2001, completing the service. LEO's outreach began with the following:

- making links with substance misuse services in order to develop skills jointly
- making links with Lambeth Housing Department and homeless people's services
- making links with the Department of Social Security and with welfare benefits advisory services (an area that proved problematic for the team)
- working with courts, barristers and solicitors on forensic matters and on issues connected with the support of clients who were refugees or asylum seekers.

I'm now taking medication. I didn't want it before but I'm accepting it. They explained it to me first, they gave me a leaflet and said why they thought I should have it. I chose the one with very little side effects.

LEO interviewee

Support groups

The idea of setting up a range of support groups grew as LEO began to work with a larger number of clients individually. With funding from the Working Together in London budget, the team began by introducing a drop-in service. This provided a safe and relaxed environment where clients could meet and decide on the activities they wanted to take part in. Team members supported the group initially, with the aim of handing over its running to the clients as they developed the confidence to take on new responsibilities. A range of activities was organised and clients taking responsibility for particular aspects of the work could be offered a small payment.

> *I go to the Thursday drop-in. It's other people with the same problems. We watch a video and sometimes talk. They organise it, but they don't tell us what we should do.*
>
> LEO interviewee

A carers' drop-in group was also set up on the same basis. Again, team members were to support the group initially, but the carers themselves would eventually take over its running. This group made links with the local Brixton Mental Health Carers group.

> *Mum knows that help is there if she needs it, but she has declined so far. LEO ask if Mum is okay and they offered her to go on a trip with other people to help them see they are not the only ones.*
>
> LEO interviewee

One interesting innovation by LEO's second team leader was a support group for gay and lesbian people with mental health problems. This has been a much-valued local resource.

Progress in partnerships

The team continued to expand its partnership work, particularly with:

- *local churches and parish workers*. Mental health services were able to raise awareness of mental health matters, and to link some clients with churches and religious groups that contributed to the network of community support.
- *the local college*. A new staff member had been recruited to support students with disabilities, and it was a real step forward to be able to incorporate mental health into other disability work; with the local Mind group, the team continued to provide the mental health awareness programme for all tutors at the college, not just those working in special needs.
- *the local Vocational Strategy Group*. LEO's development worker played an important role in this group, which addressed practical employment issues in Lambeth.

Work with black and minority ethnic communities

More than half the team's clients were from black and minority ethnic communities, and perhaps a third had arrived in the UK during the preceding four years. The needs of people from ethnic minorities are very much at the heart of LEO's work. The team was particularly conscious of the anxieties that many black people have about mental health services, and wanted to make good links with local community organisations and religious groups so that it could raise awareness of the service and listen to the community's concerns.

LEO established contact with the Fanon Project, a service for African-Caribbean people, and with Amardeep, which provides community support for Asian clients. The team's health promotion work made clients aware of organisations such as

Blackliners, which offers telephone advice, and of local support organisations such as the Black Support Group based at Brixton Road. Most African clients wished to make closer links with relevant community groups and the team was able to help them with this.

Effects on existing services

LEO appears to have caused an increase in the use of other services, and in-patient care has not as yet decreased. However, the average length of hospital stay for LEO clients is higher than the average, which suggests that only service users with the greatest needs are being admitted. As in other areas, there remain the problems of in-patients who stay for long periods and cannot be discharged and of patients who are discharged but quickly return – the so-called 'revolving door' patients.

There are cost pressures on the mental health services and the number of community posts in each sector has been reduced. Thanks to the existence of LEO, however, services have not suffered. Existing services have a long tradition of working with 'hard-to-engage' clients and lessons have been learned from the past. Funding of the LEO ward is secure, but the team is concerned that the level of funding is too low.

What has worked well

LEO has achieved some success and has become a well-regarded part of the local mental health system:

- The entire LEO service is expanding: the in-patient ward is open, the assertive outreach team is operating an 'in-reach' service for clients who need admission, and a new crisis/assessment team is being developed.
- Client engagement with the outreach team has been excellent: only one client has refused contact out of the 77 seen in the first two years.
- Client feedback is positive.
- The user drop-in and the carer support groups are both functioning well.
- Having a dedicated development worker has paid dividends: the team's clients have been able to gain access to a wide range of community services and groups – and those groups have been willing to offer support.

Partnerships have grown: with the college, with faith communities, with social services and housing, with the Fanon Centre, with the trust Arts project and with the Lambeth youth service.

> *I go to college twice a week, during the day. I do drawing and computers. LEO put me on to it. I enjoy it.*
>
> LEO interviewee

What needs improvement

> *The support workers come round when they feel like it, but [when] I wanted to speak to a support worker . . . one was on holiday and the other was off sick. They say phone whenever and then they're not there.*
>
> LEO interviewee

The team itself identified the following aspects that needed improvement:

- Working with five catchment area teams and wards has made service integration difficult; achieving this will need sustained effort.
- Team members have had problems in developing their professional roles in new ways and in coping with dual expectations from clients: for example, a psychologist working as a care co-ordinator.
- The team lost its vocational worker early on and was unable to fill the post. This has been a considerable loss, as employment is very important to the clients and other team members have been unable to provide the considerable amount of support they need to find work.
- The team has had three team leaders in three years. Each period of change has been difficult, but each new leader has contributed a distinctive strength to the work of the team.
- Substance misuse has been a major problem for the team's clients, and the team will need to make continued efforts to address this.

The future

LEO deserve a better building. It's fine for what it is, but why couldn't it be better? They deserve it.

LEO interviewee

With the end of its programme grant, LEO has received mainstream funding and is planning the following:

- to invite a team client and a carer to join the project steering group
- to further develop early onset services, establishing a community access team and OASIS, a service linked into primary care (this already exists in embryonic form but needs additional funding).
- to encourage clients to take even more control of the drop-in service, which is moving towards being user-led.

There is a regular audit of services, and the views of clients and carers are fed back.

Part three
Opportunities for
broader change

This part of the report looks at two areas where, in the interests of their clients, mental health services could be more closely involved: regeneration initiatives and faith communities.

Mental health problems are particularly common in deprived communities, and therefore mental health agencies will often be operating in the same neighbourhoods as urban regeneration programmes. Agencies should form strategic partnerships with regeneration initiatives to ensure that they take account of the needs of people with severe mental health problems.

Spirituality and religious observances are known to be very important to people with severe mental health problems. Mental health services should therefore aim to form partnerships with faith communities, which in many cases are already operating their own support systems for people with such problems.

→ CASE STUDY: SARA

Sara is a young woman who was born and brought up in London. Sara was doing well at school and enjoyed a good social life, but became worried by hearing information about her family that she hadn't known about previously. Sara was frustrated and angry that her family wouldn't discuss these matters with her and she began to experiment with drugs. This caused problems at school and at home. She became isolated and stayed in her room for long periods.

Sara's mother noticed that she was talking to herself and laughing inappropriately. She believed that people were communicating with her from the television. Later Sara attacked and injured her brother. She was taken to a police station and was admitted to hospital under the Mental Health Act, where she was diagnosed as having drug-induced psychosis. The assertive outreach team became involved around the time of planning her discharge.

After her discharge from hospital Sara wouldn't take her medication and her mother supported her in this stance. The conflict in the family continued. Sara carried on using illicit drugs and got involved with a group of other people with mental health problems who were taking drugs. She refused to engage with treatment for her serious mental health problems.

The team has maintained support for Sara and her family, offering family therapy, but she is no longer tolerated at home. The team has worked to find appropriate residential care and to ensure that education is offered in sexual health and drugs issues. The team has also worked to recognise the early signs for relapse and continues to offer Sara a range of bio-psychosocial interventions, including medication, psychological interventions and talking therapies. This is a difficult situation and one where the team will need to remain involved fully and over a long period.

7 Regeneration and mental health

The teams in Haringey, Islington and Lambeth that formed part of the Working Together in London programme were all looking to create local opportunities for change in areas where regeneration and community development had long been established. They wanted to make links that could work to the benefit of their clients and could also help the wider group of people with mental health problems in those areas.

Can urban renewal help the teams' clients?

The programme organisers used this opportunity to look at how far policies for urban and community renewal were helping people with long-term and serious mental health problems. Agencies responsible for housing, environment, education and training, and economic development are all working on programmes to tackle neighbourhood decline and social exclusion. This part of the Working Together in London programme, known as the regeneration and mental health project, was designed to establish whether this activity had had – or might in future have – a beneficial effect on mental health and mental health care.

The regeneration and mental health project therefore invited interested practitioners and policy makers to a short series of seminars to discuss how a range of policies might promote better mental health. These policies would take a 'twin track' approach: not only promoting good mental health, but also helping to improve the lives of people who had already experienced mental health problems. As with the rest of the programme, the basic aim was to enable people with mental health problems to have a decent life, with a home, some money, something worthwhile to do in the day and the opportunity to develop a network of contacts and friends.

> Helen had schizophrenia. Local children chased her, threw stones and hurt her. Helen got involved in a gardening group at the Healthy Living Centre, where she worked alongside the mothers of some of those children. They all got to know each other, the persecution stopped and Helen and the children began to swap videos. A new relationship – one of friendship – emerged in the flats where they all lived. People living in the flats later got involved in plans for the new housing.
>
> Alison Trimble, Bromley by Bow Healthy Living Centre, in King's Fund, 1999

The policies that matter

Some old policies and some newer ones might have an effect on mental health in an area. They would include:

- regeneration schemes, including the Single Regeneration Budget
- Welfare to Work
- widening participation in lifelong learning
- Health Action Zones
- the New Deal for Communities.

As we have seen, mental ill health is closely associated with unemployment, living alone in poor and insecure housing and having a low income. In addition, people who are from black and minority ethnic communities or are refugees face racism and discrimination (King's Fund, 1997). If mental health is to be improved, policies are needed that will help to remove these disadvantages.

The Working Together in London programme does not suggest that these policies would of themselves prevent people from developing mental ill health. What the programme has begun to show is that, by tackling the problem of social exclusion, the lives of people with serious and long-term ill health can be improved in the community. Improvements in the quality of life for people from disadvantaged communities can also strengthen the capacity of those communities to maintain their own good mental health.

The policies that contradict each other

For perhaps thirty years, until the publication of the *National Service Framework* (Department of Health, 1999), a major preoccupation of mental health policy was public safety. However, Standard 1 of the Framework talks of the wider determinants of mental ill health. It mentions the need to improve people's lives and combat prejudice. This has been a welcome contribution to changing the focus of policy from managing ill health to creating the conditions for good mental health.

Unfortunately, while the Framework adopts a positive approach, other influences are driving mental health policy towards maintaining its emphasis on public safety and containing the individual, the most significant example of this being the draft Mental Health Bill (Stationery Office, 2002). This contradiction will not be discussed in this review, but the impact of punitive policies on the willingness of society to work alongside people with mental health problems in the community cannot be ignored (Laurance, 2002).

Making positive connections

Despite possible setbacks in some areas of mental health policy, there are still excellent opportunities for making connections between urban regeneration programmes and mental health. To date, these opportunities have only been taken up in a limited way, but as the series of King's Fund seminars held in 1999 and 2000 showed the conditions are now right to do much more.

The priorities for making progress are:

- a source of basic information about the many policies relating to community development and urban renewal and to mental health policy – together with examples of practice linking the two
- opening a dialogue at local level to bridge the conceptual gap and to create better understanding
- building on the kind of partnership working that Working Together in London has shown can be successful
- changing the outcome measures for mental health so that they look at the quality of people's lives as well as the results of treatment
- changing the outcome measures for urban regeneration so that they check how far schemes actually deliver for people with mental health problems.

The consequences of failure will be that the most excluded people, including those with long-term mental health problems, will continue to live in isolation, their talents and potential contribution to society ignored to the continuing detriment of their mental health.

Employment

I'm supposed to be working full-time but I'm off because of physical problems, not mental health problems . . . it really kills me not to be at work. I don't take to being off work . . . I can't bear sitting and watching TV, just watching the clock and the hours go by.

LEO interviewee

There is growing evidence for the importance of work in enabling the users of mental health services to obtain a better quality of life. The quotation above shows the soul-destroying effects of having nothing to do day after day. For people whose illness may itself have brought about isolation, to be deprived of the social benefits of employment is an even greater blow.

There is also the problem of the poverty that many people with mental health problems experience. Despite all that assertive outreach and other mental health teams do to improve people's welfare benefits, in the long term their income is always going to be less than if they were in employment.

As a sick person it seems to take a lot longer. I was in hospital and I had to go with being a lone parent just to get some money. LEO helped by writing letters to the benefits agency but they [the benefits agency] didn't seem to care. I thought that was terrible.

LEO interviewee

The three Working Together in London teams have rightly identified employment as a key priority for their clients. However, each of them has found it difficult to sustain their input and each now plans to develop new approaches.

Education and training

Each of the teams has also identified the importance of education and training. These have featured particularly prominently for Antenna and LEO, as they have a somewhat younger client group. At a King's Fund seminar in 1999, New College Nottingham, a large further education college, reported the views of some of its students who have mental health problems but are supported in the mainstream college programme. They said that going to college:

> . . . gives structure to the day.
> . . . provides contacts and gives me confidence.
> . . . gives some possibilities in my life.
> . . . brings less isolation.

King's Fund, 1999

The requirements for change

Good progress has been made, both in education and training and in routes into employment (Bates, 2002):

- A variety of routes into work are now available that do not restrict the user to old-style day services – but much remains to be done to ensure that this kind of development continues.
- There is a range of employment schemes for people with mental health problems that offer routes into work and include job brokerage, mentoring and coaching to help people to keep the jobs they find.

As yet, however, not all mental health services see routes into work as being as legitimate a goal as treatment. What we need is:

- continued emphasis by local mental health policy makers on the importance of improved routes into education and training and into work
- continued attention from local partnerships for economic regeneration and employment to education and training and work for people with mental health problems
- outcome measures for mental health services and for economic development partnerships that will show what is happening for people with mental health problems who want to find work
- continued attention at national level to ensure that welfare benefits rules do not disadvantage people with mental health problems who want to work (including part-time)
- a change in the mental health services themselves so that people who are service users can become employees. Again, this is happening, but progress is slow.

> Mental illness has a great impact on the economy, costing around £12 billion a year in welfare benefits and wreaking a huge toll in disability. There is a clear association between social deprivation and mental illness . . . It is possible to reduce the incidence of mental health problems, but this has never been a priority for the NHS. This will change as the National Service Framework on mental health is implemented.

Professor Graham Thornicroft in King's Fund, 2000

Summary

■ The Working Together in London teams all operate in areas where regeneration and community development initiatives are common.

■ The programme organisers therefore ran a series of events to discuss how regeneration programmes could help people with severe mental health problems.

■ The ingredients for success were identified as: access to good information about urban renewal and mental health; close partnership working; and developing the outcome measures for both regeneration and mental health care so that they actually deliver for people with severe mental health problems.

■ Suggested actions include:
  – persuading partnerships to provide training and employment for people with severe mental health problems
  – ensuring that benefits rules do not penalise people with severe mental health problems who want to work
  – enabling former users of mental health services to become employees of those services.

8 Faith communities and mental health

What religion I do have is an important part of my life. I believe in Jesus Christ and values like love, hope and peace. I also believe in prayer. I'm an excommunicated Jehovah's Witness so don't go to a Jehovah's Witness church every week. I go to a non-denomination church. Group prayer is very important to me.

LEO interviewee

Mental health services have been slow to recognise the importance of spirituality and religious observance to many people with mental health problems – perhaps because they fear that their own lack of understanding of these matters might cause difficulties. But the situation is changing, and there is in particular a growing recognition of the importance of spirituality and religion to people from black and minority ethnic communities (Copsey, 2001).

Many people are telling us that their personal experiences of religion and spirituality are central to their lives and are central to how they handle and cope with their mental distress.

Melba Wilson in King's Fund, 2001

Learning how we can help each other

Of those who supported the setting up of the Antenna service, some of the most influential were members of the local community associated with the black Christian churches. The new team acknowledged that:

- for many people with mental health problems, spirituality and religious observance were very important and the team would need to recognise this in its dealings with clients
- faith communities were important local voluntary groups contributing to community life and supporting many people with mental health problems.

It was important to maintain good contacts on these two levels. Antenna remains linked with the local Christian churches, but as it also has clients from the Muslim community, the team has made appropriate connections in order to support them.

Similarly, the LEO development worker soon recognised that local faith groups would be important to the work of the team. However, there is a huge range of faith communities in Lambeth, and within these communities, there are many local places of worship used by clients of the team. LEO has therefore been slower to make the necessary links. However, the team continues to support individual clients in practising their faith and to work in partnership with faith communities.

I have friends through church that I can talk to.

LEO interviewee

Practical steps for building partnerships

At a King's Fund workshop held in 2001, more than a hundred people from mental health services and from black majority Christian churches came together to discuss partnership building. Some of the points that arose from their discussion are given below. There are to be further discussions centred around other faiths as the Working Together in London programme draws to a close.

A role for the faith communities

- to provide a route of access and referral to mental health services
- to continue to provide spiritual guidance, counselling and emotional support to people with mental health problems
- to support the carers and family network of people with mental health problems
- to help the mental health services to understand spiritual and religious matters, especially as they may affect people with mental health problems.

A role for the mental health services

- building partnerships with local faith communities, and recognising the importance of such partnerships to developing appropriate mental health care
- supporting local faith communities with the capacity building and sometimes the financial help they need to become partners in delivering services
- providing information and advice about mental health problems and services to ministers, religious and community leaders and lay people in local faith communities.

Where can we begin?

There is a need to improve partnerships between mental health services and faith communities. Research shows that all of the risk factors advanced for high rates of mental illness in black communities cannot account for all of the problems. We quickly see the linkage between black people's treatment in this society and mental ill health. This is linked with identity in their community and to spirituality. If communities tackle problems in collaboration with mental health services, we can work at the preventive level.

Dr Kwame McKenzie in King's Fund, 2001

There are, however, some obstacles to progress in this area. For some people, religious belief may have played a part in bringing about their mental distress, while others may have found faith communities to be unhelpful or even hostile:

I only sing at home to praise God. I don't like the preaching at church.

Islington interviewee

- Mental health services need to handle this matter with sensitivity.
- Partnership working can be time-consuming for mental health services, because there will be many different cultural and religious groups in any urban area. However, learning to communicate will pay off, as it will lead to the growth of new partnerships.
- Partnership working is also time-consuming for faith communities. Religious leaders have many commitments and lay workers often have families and work

responsibilities of their own, so initial expectations should not be pitched too high.

If partnerships are to flourish, the following first steps may be useful:

■ Mental health services and faith leaders should work together to raise awareness of mental health problems and to agree on the kind of support that may be available in the local area,
■ Mental health teams should support any client wishing to make contact with a religious group so as to take part in religious observance.
■ Faith communities may be able to identify service gaps and fill some of them: for example, by providing a befriending service.

It is important to remember that some people attribute their mental health problems to religion, and that this type of partnership working can be very time-consuming for both parties.

Summary

■ Religion and spirituality can be very important to people with severe mental health problems, but mental health services have been slow to recognise this.
■ The Working Together in London teams realised early on the importance of working with local faith communities; however, this proved difficult for LEO early on, because of the sheer number of places of worship in Lambeth.
■ A King's Fund workshop suggested that faith communities could: make referrals to mental health services; provide spiritual guidance for people with severe mental health problems; and give practical support to their carers.
■ For their part, mental health services could: build partnerships with faith communities; build the communities' capacity to contribute to the partnership; and advise members of the communities on mental health issues.

Part four
What the teams achieved

The final part of the report looks first at the evaluation of the Working Together in London programme carried out by the Sainsbury Centre for Mental Health and the Centre for the Economics of Mental Health. After a description of the aims and methods of the evaluation, there are discussions of the findings concerning:

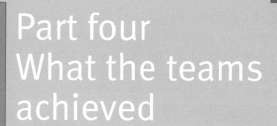

- the approach the teams took to staffing, organisational matters and service delivery
- partnership working, including steering groups and links with agencies outside mental health
- service integration.

The report concludes with detailed recommendations for policy makers and service providers on the following themes:

- promoting the social inclusion of people with mental health problems
- achieving a more integrated mental health service system
- establishing and maintaining assertive outreach teams
- listening to service users
- securing top-level commitment.

Muhammed, a 25-year-old African Muslim man, arrived in the UK two years ago seeking asylum. He lived in council accommodation in London with his three small children. In his home country, Muhammed had been an affluent man with many properties and assets. But, during political unrest, his wife was murdered and the Government seized his assets. He couldn't work due to his political status and relies on benefits such as food vouchers to support his family.

Several months ago Muhammed's children stopped going to school. Social services became involved and discovered that Muhammed was severely depressed and suffering post-traumatic stress disorder. Because of his experiences he was suspicious of psychiatric services and reluctant to engage with them. The three children moved to live with members of the extended family temporarily.

The assertive outreach team was called in and had to undertake intense social intervention to gain Muhammed's confidence and trust. He wanted his children to move back home, so the team contacted Sure Start for help with childcare issues. Muhammed started medication for depression. He found a good solicitor, who was able to help with his asylum application and he was also able to speak on his own behalf throughout his asylum process.

Muhammed continued to take medication and combined this with counselling. Eventually he stopped taking anti-depressants. He was able to regain some of his assets and now plans to return to his country next year. The assertive outreach team and Muhammed's extended family continue to support him and the children.

9 The evaluation and its findings

About the evaluation

The Working Together in London programme was evaluated by a team from the Sainsbury Centre for Mental Health (SCMH) and a team from the Centre for the Economics of Mental Health. In order to gain a fresh perspective, the SCMH team was made up of researchers who had not hitherto been involved in the programme. The staff from SCMH and the King's Fund who had selected, trained and supported the teams took no part in the evaluation.

An innovative feature of the evaluation was the inclusion of the views of users of the services themselves. The Sainsbury Centre user-focused monitoring team recruited and trained users to carry out these interviews. The views of the 21 users and four carers they spoke to form part of the evaluation.

For those who wish to see the complete findings and the economic evaluation of the teams, the full evaluation report is available on request from the Sainsbury Centre for Mental Health and the King's Fund (Lee, McCrone and Ford, 2002).

This evaluation may also be set alongside other current evaluation exercises. Three of these are related to this programme:

- Two randomised controlled trials (RCTs) on the effectiveness of the assertive outreach teams in Islington and in Lambeth. Islington is due to report late in 2004 and Lambeth late in 2003.
- The pan-London study of assertive outreach teams intends to examine specifically inner-city assertive outreach team practices against US fidelity criteria. It is hoped to learn something more about the 'critical components of assertive outreach provision in the British context' (Greatley and Ryrie, 2001). This will report in 2004.
- Readers who want to see the methodology employed and look at the details of service use and costs should obtain a copy of the full evaluation report from the King's Fund or SCMH. This chapter draws on the evaluation to explore, firstly, what local stakeholders thought about the service.

The aims

The evaluation looked at what it is about the Working Together programme that works, for whom and in what circumstances.

It investigated the following areas:

- partnership working – the level of co-operation and collaboration between key stakeholders and the extent to which this leads to the planning or introduction of initiatives that will have an impact at ground level

- service integration – identifying ways to enhance integration, including links and connections between assertive outreach and other services within the mental health system
- service user and carer views on plans for change and the prospects for integrated care
- black communities' views on plans for change and the prospects for better services for black people
- programme participants' views on whether the prospects for mental health services have improved as a result of this initiative
- the economic impact of services on users, carers and providers.

This work complements the randomised controlled trials in South Islington and Lambeth. It will also provide additional information on integration, users' views and partnerships to that contained in the pan-London study of assertive outreach teams that will be published in 2004.

The methods

Stakeholder interviews were carried out in two phases. The initial phase, between October and November 2000, involved interviews with 28 people across the three sites. The interviewees came from a variety of organisations, including local councils, the police and colleges, but they were mainly people from statutory organisations in the health and social service sectors with a primary interest in mental health. These included members of the Working Together in London teams themselves. The findings from this initial stage were reported in some detail to the programme funders and to the teams and steering groups on each site. The fact that most interviewees were from statutory mental health agencies meant that these findings were focused on the themes of team operation, the teams' integration with other local mental health services, and partnerships largely within the statutory sector.

The second stage of stakeholder interviews, carried out between June and August 2001, involved 23 individuals from non-statutory, community and voluntary sector organisations. The intention was to acquire a broader perspective on the work of the teams, and in particular to focus on social inclusion, a key part of the initial aims of the programme. It was felt that talking to agencies outside the mental health field – such as churches and leisure, training and employment organisations – would help the evaluation to examine how widely the teams had been collaborating on the social inclusion agenda.

This chapter briefly revisits some of the key findings from the first stage of interviews and then examines what the second stage of interviews add to these findings. The main themes are:

- team approach
- partnership
- integration
- social inclusion.

The approach taken by the teams

Staffing

The initial stakeholder interviews revealed that the LEO site had had some early problems in recruiting, particularly for the vocational worker post. The position was eventually filled in September 2000 after three rounds of interviews, but by the summer of 2001 this worker had left. One interviewee said:

> There was a worker employed with the team who was to concentrate on linking clients into vocational services. However, this person left and has not been replaced. The result is that clients are not getting the help they should with this.

The LEO site has also had three team leaders since it was established.

The initial project manager from the Antenna team left for promotion within the trust and the team leader at that time took over the position of project manager. An outreach worker also left Antenna for promotion and one of the nurses (F Grade) left LEO for a similar post in another assertive outreach team. A G grade nurse left the Islington team because she did not find the team approach to her liking; she preferred having an individual caseload and has gone back to working for a community mental health team.

Establishing the teams

A key focus of the initial stage of stakeholder interviews was the way in which the teams were set up. Certain key factors, identified at all three sites, were seen as contributing to success:

- *The skills, experience and commitment of team members*. There were people in each team who had previous experience of working in assertive outreach teams. The teams were also seen as being very enthusiastic, dedicated and determined to ensure that the services succeeded.
- *The support of the trust*. The local trust's commitment was seen as vital to the operation of the teams. For example, in Islington the implementation of the AO team, along with the introduction of a crisis team, was a central part of the mental health strategy that the trust had agreed with the health authority before the Working Together in London programme.
- *Training*. The training undertaken by the teams (much of it provided by the training section of the Sainsbury Centre for Mental Health) was seen as important for team building.
- *Money*. The extra funding provided by the Working Together in London programme was seen as critical in enabling the services to be established.
- *Time*. The teams were given time for training and setting up before they started seeing clients. When they did start taking referrals, the slow intake of clients was thought to have helped prevent them from being inundated, which can often happen with new services.

The medical versus the social model

Interviewees at the second stage were asked for their impressions of the teams' general approaches and the extent to which they were medically or socially focused.

There was consensus amongst the Antenna stakeholder interviews that the team had adopted a 'social' approach. This respondent from the local recreational services provided was typical when he said:

> They provide a culturally sensitive service, unlike statutory services. I would say they were definitely not medical but social in approach.

Other people made slightly different responses, with one feeling that Antenna offered a 'family orientated' service. Another referred to the way that Antenna worked as a team and was not restricted by the hierarchical structures that sometimes prevent effective team working in the statutory sector. She said:

> I think Antenna is eclectic. They have adopted an assertive outreach model of working, which is appropriate. The team does not appear to be bound by any one profession, as you often find in statutory services, but works as a team.

LEO stakeholders were more divided on this question, with most considering the team's approach to be a combination of medical and social. One stakeholder felt that although it was partly medical, the team was less rigid in its approach than mainstream mental health services were. Only two stakeholders expressed dissatisfaction with the team's approach on the grounds that it was far too medically orientated, which was against the supposed philosophy of the assertive outreach approach and not what they were set up to be. One stakeholder noted:

> LEO is definitely medical, as medication is the main issue for the team, despite the fact they were supposed to have a social rehabilitation focus. The team has been overrun with the demands of care co-ordination and care management, with its medical focus.

Most stakeholders interviewed about the Islington team felt that it too had adopted a largely medical focus. Several stakeholders had reservations about the team's philosophy, especially the emphasis it placed on clients taking their medication. A stakeholder from the local trust said:

> They are medically driven, which they shouldn't be. This is due to the fact that certain personalities, for example the psychiatrist, are too controlling. The team's main aim is to ensure clients take their medication.

Another stakeholder felt that the professional background of the workers determined whether they were medically or socially focused; support workers were more socially orientated and nurses and medical staff were medically orientated.

Taken overall, the stakeholder interviews were of the opinion that the teams' approaches occupy different positions on the spectrum between the medical and the social. It was widely agreed that Antenna had adopted a predominantly social approach. Islington, on the other hand, was seen as overtly medical – a cause for concern among some stakeholders, who felt the team was not using a true assertive outreach approach because it concentrated too much on clients taking their medication. The LEO team fell somewhere between the two positions. Some stakeholders felt that the medical aspects of the team were dominant and that it should refocus itself more towards social rehabilitation, which they felt had been a key part of its initial remit.

The impact of the teams

In the first interviews stakeholders had very high expectations of what the three teams would achieve. In the second stage of stakeholder interviews we asked respondents what they felt the impact of the teams had been so far. From their responses it would seem that the teams have gone a long way towards meeting these expectations.

At the Antenna site, in particular, the interviewees were full of praise for the work done by the team. One said:

> *Antenna is a really innovative service and it has been great to have them around . . . They do incredibly good work. They reduce the chaos in the lives of their clients, which is greatly appreciated . . . They provide what other services have so poorly failed to provide – a culturally sensitive service, which is excellent and very much needed. They are respected by the community and have developed good relationships with the local community, both clients and services.*

Another respondent said:

> *They do excellent work and we have learned a lot here from working with them. We have noticed big changes in their clients as they have progressed through the programme. When they first come here they don't look at you or speak to you, but over time you see a real change in their behaviour. Antenna can communicate with young people; they understand the issues this client group has by offering a culturally appropriate service. They might see us, as white people, as authoritarian but we can't communicate with them as Antenna can.*

Respondents at LEO were also complimentary. One interviewee said:

> *I am most impressed by their service. They provide a co-ordinated service offering, amongst other things, family support and in-patient facilities.*

Two other respondents were more reserved in their assessment of the impact of LEO, but were still generally positive:

> *They have engaged some people effectively by preventing, in particular, further deterioration of some client's mental health problems. They have 'tested the water' of the realities of working with young people and, in the process, have discovered more questions than answers.*

> *Hard to tell yet. I think they are slowly becoming more well known and that their impact will grow as they are better known.*

Assessments of the overall impact of the Islington team were also positive. Two of the interviewees said:

They have kept some people out of hospital by supporting them in the community . . . I think it is a good service, although I know that not everyone does. I have seen my clients benefit from contact with the team.

They have managed to keep some people in the community for longer. The overall frequency of admissions has also been reduced – slightly, which would seem to suggest that people are more contained in the community than they used to be.

What improvements are needed?

Respondents were also asked in what areas they thought the teams could make improvements.

As Antenna was so highly regarded, many of the suggestions from stakeholders in the area centred on the team extending its service – geographically and in terms of its referral criteria and the nature of the services it offered. One respondent suggested that Antenna should serve the whole borough. Another felt that it should see people who had more in-patient admissions than its current clients. A further suggestion was that Antenna should see other minority ethnic groups such as members of the Turkish population, who were felt to need culturally appropriate services too.

In terms of what the team does, suggestions ranged from developing a branch of the service focusing on psychological interventions to workshops on parenting skills that would educate young people in the responsibilities of having children. Several respondents also said that Antenna could do more outreach work – not only in terms of staff going out on to the streets and estates to make contact with individuals who could benefit from their service but also in terms of educating teachers and children in schools about mental health issues. The interviewees recognised, however, that any expansion of the service would require more staff and resources.

Two respondents said that the LEO service should be made more social in its approach and that the level of user involvement in the work of the team should be increased:

There needs to be more emphasis on social issues. I think it should also be more user led – clients do not have enough involvement in the day-to-day team operation.

I'd like to see them develop by having a stronger user involvement. They should also have a space where service users attend regularly and are able to help with service development. The focus should also be more social.

Other suggestions concerned the staffing of the LEO team, as in this comment:

The power dynamics of the team are a significant issue. Staff need to be nurtured, otherwise they will leave. At the moment there are unequal relationships within the team, viz. the control being medical when

*it should be more equal – as is the philosophy of the assertive
outreach model.*

Two other respondents suggested that the LEO team should promote itself more
among other organisations and young people to make sure that people are aware
of who it is and what it does.

One suggestion concerned the kind of clients the Islington team saw:

*I would like them to see clients that they should be seeing, but that they don't
tend to. What I mean by this is people who are known to them but whom they
know to be particularly hard to engage.*

Another interviewee had particular concerns over the use of in-patient beds:

*My concern is that the eight beds assigned for the assertive outreach team are
always full – how is this the case if clients seen by the team are on enhanced
care in the community? Surely the idea is to keep people out of hospital . . .
They should see their clients more often and for longer – this might help to
keep people in the community.*

A further suggestion concerned what the respondent saw as the excessively
medical focus of the Islington team:

*They should spend more time with their clients. They also need more training
around psychosocial interventions, so they are less medically driven. There
needs to be a more flexible, less medicalised regime in place. Unless they
relinquish some of their medical focus they will lose non-medical staff and just
become medical and nursing focused, which is not what an AOT should be.*

The stakeholders also suggested some improvements the teams might make. For
Antenna this could largely be summed up as 'more of the same', with interviewees
often suggesting an expansion of the service in terms of geography, number of
staff and the activities it undertook. The suggestions for the Islington and LEO
teams were more fundamental, however, with concerns being expressed about
their tendency towards an overly-medical model.

Partnership

Initial stakeholder interviews had provided information about how partnership
working was being approached in two main areas: consortiums and steering
groups, and wider partnership working.

Consortiums and steering groups

All three sites had an initial consortium of individuals from a range of statutory
and voluntary agencies along with user and carer representatives. It was from
these groups that the main focus of the Working Together in London bids emerged.
Once the bids were successful, however, the nature of the partnership groups that
replaced these initial consortiums varied at each site.

LEO had established a consortium consisting mainly of people at director level in
health, social services, the police, probation, the voluntary sector, housing and

the local Health Action Zone, together with LEO team members. The consortium meets about every six months to give feedback to LEO on what it is doing from a borough-wide perspective. There is also a steering group, which consists of managers and staff from the trust, LEO team members and those involved with the randomised controlled trial (RCT) of the service. It meets monthly and focuses more closely on the day to day operation of the service.

In Islington the relatively small membership of the steering group was drawn from trust management, the team itself and those undertaking the RCT of the service. Once the team had been established, the steering group met on an *ad hoc* basis to discuss specific issues rather than having a regular pattern of meetings.

Antenna has a steering group that meets monthly and is composed of representatives from Antenna, the trust, the health authority and the local council. The initial consortium had 25–30 members and met twice a month.

There was little comment on these groups from the second stage stakeholder interviewees, as very few of them were members or had been involved with them.

What comments there were on these groups came from interviewees at the Antenna site. One said that he had attended a couple of the steering group meetings and felt that all the people who should have been there were. He did, however, feel that there should have been a greater representation of people from Edmonton. Although it bordered Tottenham, Edmonton was in a different borough (Enfield) and was therefore often overlooked in discussions, which was frustrating to those working in the area. Another interviewee felt that employers should be involved in the Antenna steering group, as this might raise awareness of mental health and perhaps help to reduce stigma in the workplace. Yet another interviewee said that teachers should be involved, as they were in a key position to recognise needs in young people.

Wider partnership working

In the initial stage of the stakeholder interviews, we found that the teams had made contact with a wide variety of statutory and non-statutory agencies. A key aim of the second stage of interviews was to examine how far these links had led to joint working and initiatives that were likely to benefit directly the people in contact with the teams.

When we asked Antenna for a list of agencies, we found that the team had already identified potential interviewees in over 30 different organisations. There was insufficient time to interview representatives from all these organisations. From the ten organisations we did speak to, however, it was clear that effective joint working had developed. An example of this was the link with the local recreational services. Initially this was concerned with getting leisure passes for Antenna clients, but eventually involved the recreational service developing, with input from Antenna, three 12-week programmes per year of activities for Antenna clients.

Antenna clients have also been participating in activity and awareness programmes run by a local youth community support worker. The activities included sport and leisure, while the awareness work focused on drugs and violence. Antenna clients have also been referred to employment-related training in, for example, interview technique, CV writing, work placements and assistance in finding a job. A residential unit that works with 18–24-year-old men with mental health problems and prepares them for independent living by helping them with matters such as hygiene, money management and cooking skills has also taken Antenna clients.

The dedicated liaison co-ordinator from the LEO team who had the specific task of making links with a variety of agencies was able to offer us a similarly long list of the different organisations she had made contact with. LEO staff went to talk to a local college about mental health and joined the college steering group set up to think about how issues concerning people with mental health problems were handled by the college. Subsequently LEO clients have also been referred to the college to undertake courses. The representative interviewed was particularly keen to stress how supportive the LEO team had been to clients referred on to the college: for example, by accompanying them when they are interviewed for a place. LEO has also referred one of its clients to a recruitment service that helps people get back into the job market by assisting them with their CVs. The woman in question now has a job.

An example of the partnerships developed at the Islington site was the referral of clients to a voluntary sector agency that helps people with enduring mental health problems to link into training and education. The representative from this organisation was again keen to emphasise the support offered to clients by the team:

> Someone from the team always accompanies the client when they come along, which no other team does. I think this is something that is really good about them. They are also good at keeping in contact.

A contract has also been agreed with a local day centre for African-Caribbean people with mental health problems so that the people in contact with the Islington team can attend it. The centre offers daytime activities such as cookery and art. Contact has also been made with a local Irish organisation that offers counselling and psychotherapy.

It was noticeable that during the setting up of the second stage of stakeholder interviews, the Islington service was not able to identify as many contacts with agencies outside the mental health field as the other two teams. This may be explained by the differences between the respective client group: the people seen by the Islington team are older and have had more enduring mental health problems than those seen by either Antenna or LEO. This may mean that many of their clients are not yet ready to move away from specifically mental health organisations.

The relatively smaller number of partnerships developed by the Islington service may also be explained by the different structures of each of the teams. The LEO team had a dedicated liaison co-ordinator to foster links and partnerships with external organisations. Although in regular contact with colleagues, this co-ordinator did not work from the main LEO base, and thus avoided becoming too involved in day-to-day clinical matters. Antenna did not have this specific role, but much of this type of work appears to have been done by the project manager, who oversees the team but can also take on this more strategic function, while the team leader looks after the day-to-day operation of the team. The Islington team does not have separate project manager and team leader roles, and it may be that in a busy team such as this, the demands of day-to-day operational and clinical matters have monopolised the team leader's time. Many of the Islington team's links with wider organisations seem to have been made by the black and minority ethnic workers in the team, part of whose role is to develop these links.

It may be that for teams like those in the Working Together in London programme, the degree to which the role of partnership development can be separated from day-to-day operational and clinical matters is crucial. It will affect the extent to which links and partnerships can be developed into joint work that benefits clients.

Local contexts

It is important to remember that all three teams must also be judged in the context of their local area and services. All the teams were generally praised for their partnership working. For example, an interviewee in the LEO area said:

> They have been really good at making links with other organisations, and their approach should be a good model for others to follow.

The efforts at partnership working by the three teams appear all the more commendable when one considers how the stakeholder interviewees described joint working in general in each of the areas. For example, when a respondent from Antenna was asked how well local agencies worked together for people with mental health problems, he replied:

> I don't think they do in general. Different agencies can be defensive and reluctant to work with each other. There are a lot of tensions in this area between the police and statutory services, and the police and the community. The local social service department is also currently being investigated, which doesn't help . . . There is potential for services to work together if they would just sit down and communicate with each other.

Another highlighted some of the problems concerning housing touched upon in our interim report:

> I don't think agencies work together that well. Housing exclude people, these clients, and it is a huge problem. Most places do not want to take on such a difficult client group. We can help them here to lead more independent lives but then finding them suitable accommodation is extremely hard – for the above reasons.

Comments from the LEO and Islington stakeholders seemed to confirm this picture. One LEO stakeholder said:

> Agencies work quite poorly together – the left hand doesn't always know what the right hand is doing. There is often hostility from the voluntary sector towards the statutory and at the same time the statutory sector can be patronising towards the voluntary sector.

Although others at the LEO site did not paint such a bleak picture, claiming that agencies had begun to make links, they admitted that there was still a long way to go. And this was largely the view at the Islington site, where one interviewee from the voluntary sector said:

> *They work fairly well together, although there is a lot of room for improvement. I have to say that we do not always get invited to CPA meetings despite having more contact with a client than many other people invited. I think more non-medical people need to be invited to these meetings. Statutory mental health services can appear to be a bit reluctant to work with us.*

It is clear that the Working Together in London teams were operating in local areas where partnership and joint working were seen either as poorly developed or as in the early stages of development. The teams' attempts at partnership working, which were generally commended by the stakeholder interviewees, should therefore be seen within a context where joint working had not always been effective in the past.

Integration

In the initial stakeholder interviews, the teams were praised for their attempts to achieve integration with other parts of the local mental health service. This was being achieved, firstly, by going out and visiting other teams and units in the area to explain the purpose of their service and its referral or entry criteria. This had resulted in a high degree of awareness of which type of person each of the teams was designed to help.

The second aspect of integration identified was the fact that all three teams are part of their respective Trust management structures. Joint meetings for all team leaders and managers in the areas have meant that there is some form of regular contact between the assertive outreach team leaders and those of other mental health teams. This has helped to ensure that the assertive outreach teams and other local mental health services can share information about their work.

Despite this positive overall picture, the Working Together in London teams have had their problems with integration. The integration of Antenna with other formal mental health services has not been straightforward, and, in particular, involvement by social services has been limited. Although the Antenna team does include a social worker, that person is not directly managed by the social services department (SSD). Difficulties in fitting into the overall pattern of service delivery in Haringey have meant that the AO team has not always interacted with or impacted on the rest of the system. However, this is partly because Antenna targeted people who were too old for child and adolescent services and who only occasionally made contact with adult services.

One key development in Lambeth has been the recent integration of social services and health care staff in community teams. This has helped to improve communication between the different agencies. LEO draws clients from other teams in the area, but has also identified its own clients and retained them. There appears to be some perception that LEO sits outside the overall service. To avoid fragmentation, LEO may need to be brought more into the mainstream service. The aim is to transfer clients out of the LEO service within two years and for this purpose exit criteria are being drawn up.

The SSD in Lambeth pays for the social worker in the team, on whom there is quite a lot of pressure owing to the number of tribunals. Social services is concerned that, without greater integration, the social worker may become isolated from social work peers. Ideally, the team should have two social workers.

In the second stage of interviews, the accounts of integration between the assertive outreach teams and other services centred largely on joint working with individual clients and on sharing information. Most interviewees were pleased with the level of communication between the AO teams and themselves about people they had referred to their services. An Antenna stakeholder interviewee commented:

> *An Antenna staff member will come and visit a client they have on our programme, and generally gives the client a lot of support. If I ever need to ask them anything concerning a client, then they are always approachable and give good information – typically over the phone.*

LEO and Islington stakeholder interviewees both made similar comments. In addition, at both sites the Care Programme Approach (CPA) was identified as an important means of sharing information. For example, a LEO respondent said:

> *We are both involved with the client and there is a standard procedure we follow to make sure we are aware of what is going on with the client. Obviously we follow the CPA so we share information in this way.*

An Islington interviewee noted:

> *Yes, we do get feedback. Someone from the team often comes to the ward rounds, so we discuss clients then . . . We both work to the CPA and share information that way, as well as at the weekly ward reviews.*

It was clear from the second stage of stakeholder interviews that the interaction between the Working Together in London teams and other services, particularly those in the voluntary and non-mental health sectors, was good at the client level. Most interviewees were happy with the exchange of information about clients. The teams were also praised for the support they gave clients when they were referred to services seeking access to them for the first time. However, there remain concerns about the integration of the teams with mainstream mental health services in their local areas, and for Antenna concerning social services.

Randomisation

In the initial stakeholder interviews, the randomisation process associated with the randomised controlled trial (RCT) evaluations at the LEO and Islington sites was identified as a source of tension between the assertive outreach services and other mental health teams. When a person had been assessed by a member of the RCT research team and it was established that they fulfilled the entry criteria for the assertive outreach team, they were then randomly allocated either as a client of that team or as part of the control group (i.e. standard mental health services). At both sites the community mental health teams found that they referred individuals appropriately only for them to be randomised to the control group within the RCT and therefore back to the CMHT.

In the second stage of the interviews, two LEO stakeholder interviewees commented once more on the RCTs:

> *A problem I have with the referral criteria is that people are excluded at times due to the RCT. This can cause problems if the family know about referral and then the client is not accepted because LEO appears to be led by the research, which I don't think should be the case.*

> *They have a clear remit as to whom they are seeing. The only issue I have is the ethically dubious RCT and how this determines how clients are selected.*

Social inclusion

In the second stage, interviewees were asked if they felt the teams had helped their clients to achieve greater social inclusion and to gain better access to everyday services and facilities. This was a key aim of the Working Together in London initiative.

Key indicators of the extent to which the teams have brought about social inclusion are the accounts of service users in contact with the teams. There was consensus amongst the stakeholders interviewed at the second stage that the teams were making good progress on social inclusion. A respondent from the Antenna area gave a typical verdict when he said:

> *I think this is a real strength they have. They have forged excellent links with the community – linking into leisure, sports, education, etc. They develop a programme of activities to suit each client and then link them into the appropriate services. If it doesn't work, suit the client, then they don't fruitlessly pursue that programme but try something different instead.*

Similarly, another Antenna interviewee said:

> *I think they are really good at this. They devise individually tailored programmes for each client and, depending on the client's need, help link them into services.*

The LEO team was also praised by some interviewees for its work in this area:

> *They are really good at this. I know this from my own experience of them referring their clients to the college. I think they try and tailor a package to meet the needs of each individual client.*

Others were more cautious: while acknowledging that LEO had done good work in this area, they also felt there was room for improvement. This is illustrated by the following comment:

> *They need to develop this area, although there have been attempts at doing it. Particular staff members were employed with specific remits of developing these areas, e.g. vocational emphasis. However, it wasn't possible to develop specialist areas as staff became swamped with care management duties.*

There was a similarly mixed picture at the Islington site. One respondent said:

They must be good at this, as they have linked clients into our service.

However, another said:

They ideally should be doing this and I think they are, but it is still an area they could improve on.

A specific function of the black and minority ethnic workers employed in the Islington team was to improve access to mainstream services and facilities. When interviewed, one of these workers felt that the team was beginning to make progress:

One of our clients is doing very well. Through support she is going back to studying pharmacy . . . she has been going to the library and doing research work for college. She is going back to college where she started.

She also talked about their attempts to link clients from different cultures to their own community groups. For example, she has been able to link one client originally from Monserrat with the Monserrati Association. When the client had a relapse, members of the association came to visit him in hospital.

In general, then, there was a clear perception by stakeholder interviewees that the teams were making progress in social inclusion.

Summary

The approach taken by the teams

- *Staffing*. Antenna has experienced some high staff turnover; LEO has had three team leaders and persistent difficulties in recruiting a vocational worker and Islington has been concerned by potential staff 'burnout'.
- *Establishing the teams*. Key factors for success were: the skills, experience and commitment of the team members; the support of the local trust; the training provided by the SCMH; the funding supplied by the Working Together in London programme, and a generous time scale.
- *Medical versus social*. The consensus was that Antenna adopted a social approach, the Islington team a more medical one and LEO a combination of the two.
- *Impact*. All three teams were praised for their approach.
- *Improvements*. Respondents said that: Antenna should extend its service, and send more of its workers out onto the streets; the Islington team should see its clients more often and for longer; and LEO should adopt a more social approach and have more user involvement.

Partnership

- *Consortiums and steering groups*. Antenna has a steering group that meets monthly and consists of people from the team itself, the trust, the health authority and the local council; the Islington team has a relatively small steering group that meets on an *ad hoc* basis and consists of people from the team itself, the trust and the research team; and LEO has a consortium group, which meets twice yearly and consists of people at director level from local agencies, and a steering group, which meets monthly and consists of people from the team itself, the trust and the research team.

■ *Wider partnership working*. Antenna has working relationships with more than 30 organisations; they were formed by the project manager, while the team leader looked after day-to-day operations. Thanks to its dedicated liaison co-ordinator, LEO also has links with a wide range of organisations. But the Islington team has formed fewer partnerships – perhaps because it does not have a dedicated co-ordinator or separate team leader and project manager roles.

■ *Local contexts*. All three teams were operating in areas where partnership working was either poor or in its early stages of development. Therefore the teams' efforts at forming partnerships (see above) were generally applauded.

Integration

■ *Trust management structures*. Islington and LEO were part of their respective trust management structures; Antenna is a voluntary organisation, but was linked into the management structure. Therefore all three teams had regular contact with other mental health teams.

■ *Joint working*. All three teams were praised for their joint working over individual clients and for their sharing of information.

■ *Integration*. However, Antenna has not integrated fully with the other mental health services (especially the SSD) – perhaps because the people it targets are too old for child and adolescent services and do not use adult services.

■ *The mainstream service*. Similarly, LEO finds itself rather outside the mainstream service, and may need to be moved closer in order to avoid fragmentation.

■ *Randomisation*. The randomised control trial evaluations at the LEO and Islington sites were a source of tension between the assertive outreach teams and the other mental health teams.

Social inclusion

■ *Improved social inclusion*. All three teams have made good progress in improving the social inclusion of their clients.

10 Conclusions and recommendations

Assertive outreach has now become a national priority. Targets have been set for the development of teams, and there has been a rapid growth in their numbers nationally. This review has summarised the progress made in three areas of London. It has also described the opportunities that assertive outreach and other mental health teams can exploit, looking at the impact on the wider system of mental health services and on the quality of life of people with serious mental health problems.

The review gives initial findings on team development for those who are still in the early stages of their own local programme. It also looks at ways of improving the lives of people with serious mental health problems. It offers commissioners, managers and service users some insights into what worked well and what worked less well for the Working Together in London teams and suggests positive steps that might be taken on the basis of the teams' experience and the views of their clients. The review is intended to contribute to the continuing discussion on how best to implement this important development in mental health care.

The Working Together in London development programme had three key aims:

- to promote social inclusion for people with serious mental health problems
- to work within the local system of mental health services to bring about better integration of those services
- to establish three assertive outreach teams, focusing on people with the most serious problems and maintaining the work beyond the life of the programme.

The programme functioned in a very challenging environment for mental health care:

- within very deprived communities
- in areas with some of the highest levels of need for mental health care in the country
- in areas with spiralling demand for mental health services
- within complex service systems that already offered a variety of options for care.

The work of the three teams and their local steering groups was monitored regularly, and much of the material reported here has been drawn from monitoring reports as well as from the findings of the two-stage evaluation. Overall findings have already been fed back to the teams, and many of their own comments and conclusions are incorporated below.

The review shows that each of the teams enjoyed a degree of success in meeting all three aims and that there are significant opportunities to build upon this success for the future. Three main groups of findings emerged from the review. They concern:

- social inclusion
- integrating mental health care
- establishing assertive outreach teams.

Promoting the social inclusion of people with mental health problems

Many people with serious mental health problems encounter considerable obstacles when trying to achieve a better quality of life. Service users told us that they see their ordinary lives as a maze in which they are blocked at every turn, over money, accommodation, work and other practical matters.

The teams in this programme focused on issues such as housing, welfare benefits, education and training and employment to make sure that their clients could gain greater independence and achieve that better quality of life. They treated mental health problems but also supported people in getting out of the maze and becoming more able to cope.

Developing partnerships

The teams tackled these issues by developing partnerships with agencies outside traditional mental health services. The three case studies show the degree of success each team achieved through these new partnerships.

It was important for each team to be clear about its specific client group, drawn from among people with serious mental health problems. Teams were able to focus on developing partnerships to achieve what their specific clients wanted: to get and keep a home, to go back to college, to train for a job, to have some money and to go out with friends. For Antenna and LEO, education, training and leisure activities were particularly important, as they had a younger client group. For the Islington team, with its generally older client group, the need for housing and for improved welfare benefits took on a higher priority.

New opportunities for people with serious mental health problems

However, the programme was not just about the needs of the clients of these three assertive outreach teams. The teams and their local 'promoters', the steering groups, also took on the challenge of developing partnerships that could work to the advantage of any local service users who had serious and long-term mental health problems. The college that was ready to support LEO's clients has now recognised its role in supporting other people with mental health problems. The Haringey leisure service that supported Antenna's clients now understands more about opening up its provision to young people experiencing the onset of mental health problems. All these developments are in their very early stages, but they have already helped to increase social inclusion.

However, there are many agencies and services that the teams were unable to make close contact with during the life of the programme. It is not easy to identify the right agencies, services and groups and then to work with them systematically to develop partnerships. Islington's work with the very wide range of local black and minority ethnic communities has taken time to develop, but will be important for people from those communities who experience serious mental health problems. The programme has shown that new opportunities exist for partnerships with regeneration and neighbourhood renewal initiatives and with faith communities if mental health services are prepared to take a lead.

Designated staff

Teams were particularly successful in initiating and developing new partnerships where the task was taken forward by staff who worked with the team but did not carry caseloads. In the one case the project leader and in the other a development worker were able to sustain partnership working for their clients and potentially for other people with mental health problems. They were also able to make new relationships with community groups outside the mental health field. This is particularly important for promoting awareness of mental health problems and the role of mental health services in the community. Relationships with traditional churches and with a variety of faith communities showed the potential for future development that can arise from such contacts.

The case studies show that:

■ It may be difficult to build relationships with agencies unused to thinking about people with serious mental health problems.
■ It takes sustained effort on the part of mental health teams to maintain and develop partnerships.
■ Mental health services must give priority to this aspect of their work, as it is very important for people with serious mental heath problems.
■ Some groups in the community can be suspicious of mental health services and services need to work with them to break down such barriers.

 ## Recommendations to primary care trusts, strategic health authorities and mental health trusts

Standard 1 of the National Service Framework concerns mental health promotion and combating discrimination; it has provided an important impetus to tackling exclusion, but it is still limited in scope.

■ Developing partnerships with local agencies outside the mental health field must be specified as part of the mainstream work of mental health services.
■ Commissioners should give priority to developing and sustaining partnerships with housing agencies, welfare benefits service and advice agencies and education and training providers.
■ Partnership working must be properly resourced and there should be a dedicated community development worker in each assertive outreach team.

Additional recommendations to mental health trusts

Community support can make the work of an assertive outreach team more acceptable.

- Mental health services need to engage with community groups and offer them support – information, training and joint working as well as grant aid; this is particularly important for people from black and minority ethnic communities.
- Mental health services need to participate in the planning and implementation of regeneration and neighbourhood development initiatives, both to advance the interests of people with known mental health problems and to promote new ways of thinking about mental health in the community.
- Faith communities are already a source of support for people with mental health problems and should be drawn in to work with the mental health services.

Achieving a more integrated mental health service system

The second of the programme's aims was to work with existing mental health services to bring about a more integrated response for users. The assertive outreach teams had to be introduced in a way that would:

- avoid confusion for service users
- avoid further fragmentation in service response
- contribute to a better-integrated service response.

All the teams worked hard at integration with other local mental health services. However, a number of tensions had to be managed to prevent confusion and fragmentation.

Impact on service integration

Early efforts to achieve a co-ordinated response to potential users were slow, because existing teams were uncertain about how assertive outreach would affect their work and their clients. Therefore they were sometimes reluctant to refer clients, meaning that some people who might have benefited from the service remained in other parts of the system. However, members of the assertive outreach teams made it part of their early development to meet other people in the mental health services to explain their functions and their approach. This was welcomed by stakeholders in the comments reported in the evaluation.

At the time, difficulties arose in developing good working relationships with other services. For LEO there were problems over integrating its work with that of other mainstream mental health services, for Antenna there were early difficulties with social services. Clearly, any new service will have to spend time explaining its role and learning more about the work of other teams within the health and social care systems. For assertive outreach, the rapid pace of development and the persistence of disagreements about the value of the approach makes it critical that this relationship-building be undertaken early on to avoid later difficulties. Managers within each mental health service system need to identify the likely 'pressure points' and set out to minimise them.

Impact on take-up of other services

Evaluation of each of the services showed that there had been an increase in the use of hospital beds during the life of the programme. There was also continued pressure on other community mental health services, although it was thought that the focus of the work of other teams might have shifted. In Islington, for example, it was suggested that the community mental health teams had been able to work more closely with primary care. It was difficult to be certain about the reasons for increased bed use, partly because the programme was relatively short but also because evaluators could not isolate other factors that might have contributed to the increase.

It was suggested that the increase in hospital bed use might have been part of a more general trend. In addition, it was noticeable that the assertive outreach teams had engaged certain people who were otherwise outside the mental health system and for whom admission was necessary for treatment and care. It was also suggested that the end of the programme might have been too soon to see changes in the mental health and lives of people with longstanding and complex problems. However, if the costs of high quality assertive outreach services are to be met from local mental health economies, there needs to be a better understanding of the effect on other services and of how to develop support systems – such as better housing support – that will reduce reliance on in-patient care. It is known that some clients of assertive outreach will continue to need admission from time to time. However, over time these admissions may arise less frequently as a result of unforeseen emergencies, while lengths of stay decrease and discharge planning improves.

The impact of research

Other effects on the local mental health system emerged from the evaluation. The case studies show that the randomised controlled trials at two of the sites created some unexpected additional difficulties early on in the programme. Other mental health services, particularly the community mental health teams, referred clients who were thought likely to benefit from assertive outreach. However, despite their suitability, half were allocated back to 'standard care' in order to meet the requirements of the research programme. This was initially a source of tension between teams, but was later understood and accepted. However, it raised questions for people outside the mental health services, as may be seen from some comments offered in the evaluation. Managers of mental health services will wish to support research projects, but they must identify the problems that may be caused to service delivery and attempt to minimise them.

Working with primary care

Engagement with general practice to maximise referrals to assertive outreach proved difficult. Several reasons were advanced for this:

- The specialist nature of the service meant that any one practice would have few patients who might benefit from assertive outreach.
- The long-standing isolation of some people with serious mental health problems meant that they might not be known to primary care.

- GPs could be reluctant to identify some younger people as having a potentially serious and long-term mental illness.
- The RCTs might deter GPs from referral.

Neither evaluation nor monitoring was able to cast further light upon this question. It may be more important, early on, for assertive outreach teams to develop an understanding of their contribution with PCTs and to take advice about the best way to make contact with GPs and their staff.

Recommendations to mental health trusts and assertive outreach teams

Assertive outreach teams should give early priority to forming working relationships with existing mental health services (including in-patient teams), with other new teams (such as crisis resolution) and with primary care. They should aim to develop an approach that will, over time, reduce reliance on expensive in-patient beds for crisis admissions and for lengthy hospital stays.

- A local communications programme is needed early on to advise on the functions and potential of any new teams – assertive outreach, crisis resolution or early intervention – and on how their work will relate to existing services.
- Arrangements for referral and for the acceptance of clients must be agreed with existing services, in particular the speed and nature of the referral process.
- Assertive outreach teams must monitor the use of in-patient beds by their clients and plan to change the nature of these admissions over time.
- The possible effects of research intervention need to be assessed at the beginning of a programme and explained within the mental health system. Monitoring systems should identify unintended effects so that these can be tackled.
- In order to maximise referrals from primary care, assertive outreach teams will need to explain to PCTs what their role, functions and potential are.

Establishing and maintaining assertive outreach teams

The third and final aim of the programme was to establish and maintain assertive outreach teams in the three Working Together in London areas. The teams were to:

- retain their focus on the designated client group – people with serious mental health problems who do not engage with services
- meet the key criteria for assertive outreach as described in *Keys to engagement*.

The case studies and evaluation show the successes and difficulties the teams experienced in getting started and developing their services.

Recruitment and training

If a new team is to develop properly, it must set aside sufficient time for appointments and training. To be effective, this must be planned in the light of other changes happening in the local health and social care system. The three teams were set up at a time of considerable changes to services in each of the three areas. This is hardly unusual: health services, including mental health services, are subject to frequent organisational change. However, for LEO, the reconfiguration of the trust did slow down the establishment of the team. The other teams also experienced some difficulties in recruitment, but were not caught up in as major a reorganisation as LEO.

Valuing existing services

Whenever a new way of working is introduced, arrangements must be made to cover existing services. The new teams may attract staff from these services, causing yet further shortages in areas where recruitment may already be a problem. In the case of the Working Together in London programme, some members of established community teams felt that they were being put under additional strain as their colleagues moved to join the assertive outreach services. Both the new and the existing teams need development support to cope with changes in their roles and responsibilities.

There is a further problem, arising from how the new teams are perceived by the staff who remain in the existing services. When the old asylums closed, it was often difficult to maintain the services that had remained within the hospitals, because staff left to join the community teams then being set up. The practical problems of cover were complicated by the perceptions of staff in the large hospitals that their work was valued less highly than that of the new teams. A similar process may be happening now as staff join new kinds of team and leave the existing community services.

Mental health services can only be effective if all their components function properly. Managers need to plan for the development of existing services too, if the staff who remain are to feel that their work is valued.

Multi-disciplinary teams

All three teams were able to recruit staff from a broad range of disciplines. A range of backgrounds and skills is important because assertive outreach teams need to be able to engage clients from a range of cultures and backgrounds. Having once secured that engagement, teams need to be able to offer treatment, care and support that will help clients to become more independent and to manage their own mental health. Although there was some delay in recruitment, stakeholders valued the breadth and experience of the teams once they began work.

Specialist inputs

As the teams developed, they came to realise the importance of incorporating more specialist skills into their work. For Islington, the expertise required to support people with dual diagnosis was important. Vocational skills became a priority for the other teams. As assertive outreach teams mature, they will recognise where they need additional support within the team. Developments in the way that assertive outreach is used must be appropriate to the particular area in which teams work and to the team focus agreed by local stakeholders.

Response to cultural diversity

Cultural sensitivity was important to all the teams. All were committed to addressing the needs of clients from black and minority ethnic communities, but they tackled this in different ways. The staff of Antenna is African and African-Caribbean and works with young black people. This approach was highly valued by the clients. The other two teams took slightly different approaches to learning how best to work with clients from black and minority ethnic communities. For two of the teams it was also important to understand and work with youth culture if their clients were to fulfil their aspiration to live the same kind of life as their peers. How a team responds to cultural diversity is a very important matter that must be agreed within the local mental health community, so that the team can work with a clear focus.

Medical approach or social approach?

The approaches taken by the teams were characterised according to how far they were 'medical' and how far 'social'. Stakeholders in each of the areas commented on this question: Antenna was seen as following a social model, Islington was regarded as being closer to the medical model and LEO was something of a combination. Assertive outreach teams have to span both these models. They must offer social rehabilitation and support to enable clients to recover, but they must also offer expert treatment and a range of clinical interventions to sustain recovery. It may be that a team's approach initially reflects the nature of its client group: for example, medication management was seen as a top priority for older users with very long-term problems, whereas the teams working with younger people were able to focus more quickly on care and support. However, as teams mature they will need to balance their approach and match it to the aspirations of their clients.

However teams manage the medical/social balance, it is clear that they must avoid a coercive and controlling approach. The clients in our study spoke highly of how all the teams managed medication. The emphasis on education and choice rather than coercion was highly valued, as was the approach taken to engagement. Assertive outreach teams can be seen as intrusive, checking up on people and controlling their lives. However, the majority of clients interviewed for our study did not feel that the teams had operated in this way. Clearly, teams must get their approach right if they are to avoid being seen as controlling and if they are to support their clients to become independent and able to manage their own lives.

Good practice in assertive outreach

There is controversy about the degree to which an assertive outreach team should conform to certain prescribed patterns. This debate about 'real' assertive outreach or 'fidelity to the model' was current throughout the period when the three teams were being set up and continues to this day. Antenna, South Islington and LEO were established in line with the broad principles set out in *Keys to engagement*. Evaluation shows that all the teams:

- maintained focus on people with severe and long-term problems
- successfully engaged with clients
- offered frequent and intense contact

- offered a range of effective treatment options
- ensured an out of hours response (although they did not provide 24-hour team working)
- worked with users in their own homes and other 'real life' locations, avoiding office-based practices
- maintained small caseloads
- worked to improve the quality of life for clients.

However, one team felt that lack of clarity about the team approach versus keyworking might have contributed to staff burn-out. To avoid continuing problems, it is essential to be clear about this question from the establishment of an assertive outreach team.

 ## Recommendations to mental health trusts, voluntary sector providers and assertive outreach teams

Plans to set up new teams should be realistic if the considerable investment they represent is not to be lost by failure at a later stage. Trusts should:

- allocate time and resources for recruitment and team training
- provide development support for both new and existing teams
- recruit from a range of disciplines initially but re-balance skills and experience within the team as it works towards meeting the needs of its target group.

Assertive outreach teams:

- must be able to offer a full range of bio-psycho-social interventions if clients are to engage with services, receive high-quality and up-to-date treatment and improve their quality of life
- may need additional specialist resources (such as in dual diagnosis) to complement, rather than replace, the work of other team members
- should work to prescribed standards, but can adapt their approach to conform to local cultural norms
- should have a clear understanding about the balance between the medical and the social approaches and about team organisation if their staff are to achieve sustainable working arrangements.

Listening to service users; securing top-level commitment

Assertive outreach teams are now an important part of modern mental health services. Across the country, teams are developing at different rates and with different foci. Some mature teams are closely involved in supporting the growth of newer teams, and we hope that the experience of the Working Together in London teams, as described in this review, can add to the shared learning.

A rapid increase in the number of teams across the country is needed, and this will require major investment. Government must play its part by recognising the potential costs of continued reorganisation and bringing greater consistency to mental health policy. As development continues, the initial investment must be seen to be well spent.

Assertive outreach offers treatment, care and support to people with mental health problems, but must always work to ensure that they become independent and able to cope. The clients of the three services described here, and analysed in greater detail in the evaluation, offer their commentary on how assertive outreach can work well. At its best, it can enable clients to achieve that greater independence and to manage their own mental health with expert support.

Mental health communities – the primary care trusts, the trusts, the social services departments – need to give assertive outreach teams top-level support if they are to succeed. This review shows that, with that kind of support and with strong community links, it is possible to provide services that can help people with serious and long-term mental health problems to recover and to achieve greater independence.

References

Bates, P (ed) (2002). *Working for inclusion: making social inclusion a reality for people with severe mental health problems*. London: Sainsbury Centre for Mental Health.

Burns, T, and Firn, M (2002). *Assertive outreach in mental health: a manual for practitioners*. Oxford: Oxford University Press.

Copsey, N (2001). *Forward in Faith: an experiment in building bridges between ethnic communities and mental health services in East London*. London: The Sainsbury Centre for Mental Health.

Davis, A, and Hill, P (2001). *Poverty, social exclusion and mental health in the UK 1978–2000*. London: Mental Health Foundation.

Department of Health (1998). *Modernising mental health services: safe, sound and supportive*. London: Department of Health.

Department of Health (1999). *The National Service Framework for mental health: modern standards and service models for mental health*. London: Department of Health.

Department of Health (2000). *The NHS Plan: a plan for investment, a plan for reform*. London: The Stationery Office.

Department of Health (2001). *The mental health implementation policy guide*. London: Department of Health.

Department of Health (2002). *Dual diagnosis good practice guide*. London: Department of Health.

Dixon, L (2000). 'Assertive Community Treatment: twenty-five years of gold', *Psychiatric Services (a journal of the American Psychiatric Association)*, 51, 6.

Drake, R, *et al* (2001). 'Implementing dual diagnosis services for clients with severe mental illness', *Psychiatric Services (a journal of the American Psychiatric Association)*, 52, 4.

Dunn, S (1999). *Creating accepting communities: report of the Mind inquiry into social exclusion and mental health problems*. London: Mind.

Greatley, A, and Ryrie, I (2001). 'Reach out and join up', *Health Services Journal*, 111, 5759, 14 June.

Johnson, S, *et al*. (eds) (1997). *London's mental health*. London: The King's Fund.

Laurance, J (2002). 'Pure Madness: How fear drives the mental health system'. King's Fund lecture, Faculty of Public Health Medicine Annual Scientific Conference 2002. Available online at www.kingsfund.org.uk

Minghella, E, Gauntlett, N, and Ford, R (2002). 'Assertive outreach: does it reach expectations?', *Journal of Mental Health*, 11, 1, 27–42.

King's Fund (1997). *Transforming health in London: report of King's Fund London Commission*. London: The King's Fund.

King's Fund (1999). *Regeneration and mental health: briefing 2*. London: The King's Fund.

King's Fund (2000). *Regeneration and mental health: briefing 3*. London: The King's Fund.

King's Fund (2001). *Building partnerships – mental health services and the faith communities: briefing 1*. London: The King's Fund.

Lee, J, McCrone, P, and Ford, R (2002). *Independent and able to cope*. London: The King's Fund/The Sainsbury Centre for Mental Health/Centre for the Economics of Mental Health.

McGrew, J, Bond, G, Dietzen, L, and Salyers, M (1994). 'Measuring the fidelity of implementation of a mental health program model', *Journal of Consulting and Clinical Psychology*, 62, 4, 670–78.

Marshall, M, *et al* (1999). 'PriSM psychosis study', *British Journal of Psychiatry*, 175, 501–03.

Marshall, M, and Lockwood, A (1998). *Assertive Community Treatment*. Cochrane Review. Oxford: The Cochrane Library.

Phillips, A, *et al* (2001). 'Moving Assertive Community Treatment into standard practice', *Psychiatric Services (a journal of the American Psychiatric Association)*, 52, 6.

The Sainsbury Centre for Mental Health (1998). *Keys to engagement*. London: The Sainsbury Centre for Mental Health.

The Sainsbury Centre for Mental Health (2002). *Breaking the circles of fear: a review of the relationship between mental health services and African and Caribbean communities*. London: The Sainsbury Centre for Mental Health.

Sayce, L, and Measey, I (1999). 'Strategies to reduce social exclusion for people with mental health problems', *Psychiatric Bulletin*, 23, 65–67.

Stationery Office (2002). *Draft Mental Health Bill. Cm 5538 1-111*. London: The Stationery Office.

Stein, L, and Santos, A (1998). *Assertive Community Treatment of persons with severe mental illness*. New York: Norton.

Thornicroft, G, *et al* (1998). 'Ten papers from the PriSM study', *British Journal of Psychiatry*, 173, 363–427.